QuickStudy®

for

Nursing

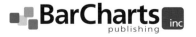

Boca Raton, Florida

©2007 BarCharts, Inc.
ISBN 13: 978-142320270-7
ISBN 10: 142320270-8

BarCharts® and QuickStudy® are registered trademarks of BarCharts, Inc.

Author: Deborah Raines, Ph.D., R.N.
Artist: Andrea Hutchinson
Publisher:

> BarCharts, Inc.
> 6000 Park of Commerce Boulevard, Suite D
> Boca Raton, FL 33487
> *www.quickstudy.com*

Printed in Thailand

Contents

Study Hints

NOTE TO STUDENT:
Use this QuickStudy® booklet to make the most of your studying time. For easier reference, most of the information in this booklet is set in table format.

QuickStudy® Nursing Notes provide need-to-know information; read them carefully to better understand key concepts. Refer to them often to avoid problems.

NURSING NOTES
The professional nurse uses all acquired skills in combination—**assessment, observation, intuition, diagnosis, planning, evaluation, documentation**—to provide the most effective nursing care for every patient.

Take your learning to the next level with QuickStudy®!

Introduction

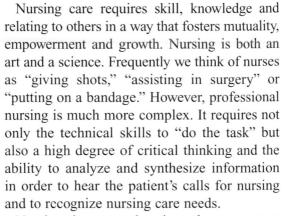

Nursing care requires skill, knowledge and relating to others in a way that fosters mutuality, empowerment and growth. Nursing is both an art and a science. Frequently we think of nurses as "giving shots," "assisting in surgery" or "putting on a bandage." However, professional nursing is much more complex. It requires not only the technical skills to "do the task" but also a high degree of critical thinking and the ability to analyze and synthesize information in order to hear the patient's calls for nursing and to recognize nursing care needs.

Nursing is more that just the competent completion of a series of tasks. Nursing is about coming to know another person within the context of a professional and caring-based helping relationship. Nursing practice requires professional judgment and critical thinking, combined with the technologic "how to" use of the materials. It is the use of cognitive technologies and critical analysis and synthesis that leads to the experiential knowledge—knowing when, how, why and what next about the material technology—that is the science of nursing practice. The art of nursing practice comes when empathic caring blends with practical skills and scientific know-how.

Introduction

Nursing Process

Assessment

The first phase of the nursing process, **assessment**, is the collection of patient-specific information for analysis and evaluation of the patient's conditions. The professional nurse is responsible for the completeness and accuracy of the information.

Types of Assessment

Determined by patient needs, time available and purpose of data collection:

Type	Focus	Example
Initial or Admission Assessment	To evaluate the patient's health status, identify problems and provide an in-depth comprehensive database. Provides a baseline to evaluate changes in the patient health status.	Patient admitted to a health-care facility
Focused Assessment	Data about a previously identified problem. Narrow in scope, focused on the specific problem's status: i.e., better, unchanged or worse.	Checking the circulation and neurological sensation of a casted extremity

Type	Focus	Example
Time-Lapsed Assessment	Reassessment of a known program/condition after the passage of a substantial period of time. Compares current status with baseline or standardized norms.	Developmental assessment of infants and children
Emergency Assessment	Priority is preservation of life. Rapid identification and intervention often focused on physiological alterations in airway, breathing and circulatory status. Psychosocial alterations involving suicidal thoughts or violent acts also initiate an emergency. Very focused but not comprehensive.	Traumatic injury

Assessment Skills

Using knowledge of nursing, basic and social sciences, and pathophysiology, nurses assess patients in sophisticated ways and with comprehensive methods, including:

■ **Observation**
   ◆ Begins when the nurse meets the patient.
   ◆ Uses all the senses, as the nurse sees, hears, smells and touches the patient.
   ◆ Involves the skill of noticing patient cues.

■ **Interviewing**
  ◆ Interaction process for gathering data through questioning and information exchange.
■ **Physical Examination**
  ◆ Using techniques of inspection, palpation, percussion and auscultation to analyze bodily functions.
■ **Intuition**
  ◆ Use of insight, instinct and/or clinical experience to make judgments about patient care.

Assessment Activities

■ **Collecting Data**
  ◆ Compiling information about the person as patient.
■ **Subjective Data**
  ◆ Symptoms or indications experienced by the patient. Includes the patient's feelings, statements, thoughts and experiences about his/her health.
  ◆ Obtained through interviewing and listening to the patient.
  ◆ Best recorded as direct quotations.
  ◆ Examples include: values, perceptions, feelings, attitudes, beliefs and symptoms.
■ **Objective Data**
  ◆ Signs or external cues that are observable and measurable.
  ◆ Obtained through the use of nurse's senses, measuring devices, equipment, laboratory studies and/or diagnostic procedures.
  ◆ Examples include: physical findings such as skin color, vital signs, heart sounds and laboratory results.

■ **Recording Data**
- ◆ Systematically placing the data into the medical record.
- ◆ Institutions have forms for recording data and facilitating use of data among providers.
- ◆ Use direct quotes to communicate the patient's perspectives.
- ◆ Use observable, measurable, specific terms to record objective data.

■ **Validating Data**
- ◆ Confirming the accuracy of the collected data.
- ◆ Compare collected data to normal function and individual patient variations.
- ◆ Check for consistency of collected data.
- ◆ Clarify patient's statements.
- ◆ Seek consensus with colleagues.

■ **Organizing Data**
- ◆ Using a framework as a guide to protect against omission of pertinent information.
- ◆ Organizing frameworks include:
  - • **Functional health patterns** that use 11 functional health patterns basic to nursing:
    - > **Head-to-Toe Model:** Systematic examination of every part of the body, starting from the head and progressing down to the toes.
    - > **Body Systems Model:** Organized examination of major anatomical systems to collect data about past or present condition of each organ or body system. Also know as the **medical model.**
    - > **Conceptual Frameworks:** Orem's self-care model, Roy's adaptation model, Neuman's system model and Johnson Behavioral model are some examples. Each has a frame of reference for organizing patient data.

Nursing Diagnosis

■ Nurses analyze and interpret the collected data resulting in a nursing diagnosis.

■ Registered nurses are licensed to make nursing diagnoses and have a duty to plan care for patients based on the identified nursing diagnosis.

Diagnosis Activities

■ **Identifying Patterns:** The collected data, subjective symptoms and objective signs are analyzed to identify patient conditions.

◆ **Cues:** Pieces of data collected during the assessment process.

◆ **Clustering:** Putting together cues that if viewed separately would not convey the same meaning; putting the pieces of the puzzle together.

◆ **Interpreting:** Synthesizing the cluster to see the whole picture and, by looking at the patterns, derive meaning or a diagnosis.

■ **Validating Diagnosis:** Corroborates the diagnosis and its significance to the patient.

Outcome Identification

■ Measurement criteria for outcome identification, which includes specifying intermediate and long-term outcomes that focus on health promotion, health maintenance or health restoration.

■ Nurse-sensitive patient outcomes and indicators demonstrate to the public how nursing achieves patient outcomes.

Establishing Priorities
■ Decision-making process of ranking the order of nursing diagnoses in terms of order of importance:
  ◆ **High Priority**
    • Life-threatening situations
    • Situations requiring immediate attention
    • Issues of importance to the patient
  ◆ **Medium Priority**
    • Anything that could result in unhealthy consequences, but that does not threaten life.
  ◆ **Low Priority**
    • Anything that is easily resolved with minimal intervention and little potential for causing dysfunction.

Establishing Goals & Outcome Criteria
■ **Goal**
  ◆ Hypothesis about the patient's state after receiving nursing care.
  ◆ Developed based on nursing knowledge and experience and in collaboration with the patient.
■ **Outcome Criteria**
  ◆ Realistic, measurable and specific statements of goal achievement.

Planning
The development of nursing care strategies to address the patient's problems.

Planning Activities
■ **Nursing Interventions:** Activities based on nursing knowledge and clinical judgment to enhance patient outcomes.
  ◆ **Types of Interventions**
    • **Psychomotor** (positioning, inserting)

- **Psychosocial** (encouraging, supporting
- **Educational** (teaching, demonstrating)
- **Maintenance** (providing, assisting)
- **Surveillance** (monitoring, detecting)
- **Supervisory** (delegating, collaborating)
◆ **Types of Plans of Care:** Consistent elements are the nursing diagnosis, patient goal and interventions; format of the plan of care may vary.
  - **Individual plan of care:** Specifically written for each patient by the nurse.
  - **Standardized plan of care:** Written by groups of nurses for a patient population with a specific diagnosis.
  - **Generic plan of care:** A plan written to a specific nursing diagnosis but then individualized to each patient's needs.
  - **Computerized plan of care:** Computer-generated and based on entered assessment data.

Implementation

The actual providing of nursing care, which requires competence in the technical, interpersonal and cognitive dimensions of nursing.

Technical Dimension

■ Helping patients retain a state of health, prevent deterioration of physical and psychological function, and preserve their independence.

■ Monitoring patient status to detect changes from baseline conditions.

■ Using skill expertise such as inserting, removing, changing, administering, or other psychomotor actions including management and care of equipment, treatments and procedures.

Interpersonal Dimension

■ Acting as a patient advocate, making referrals, collaborating with others, and maintaining a therapeutic schedule for the patient.

■ Using therapeutic communication techniques, relieving spiritual distress, and showing caring to provide comfort and healthy responses.

■ Resolving psychological, emotional or social tribulations.

Cognitive Dimension

■ Applying principles of the teaching and learning process.

■ Delegating specific aspects of care and supervising other members of the health-care team.

Evaluation

■ A judgment of the effectiveness of nursing care to meet patient goals based on the patient's behavioral response.

■ In addition to being a distinct phase, evaluation is ongoing throughout the nursing process.

Evaluation Skills

■ **Standards of Care**
   ◆ Authoritative statements made by nursing organizations, external organizations or health-care institutions.
   ◆ These statements guide nursing practice and provide the minimum standard to which nurses are held accountable.

■ **Normal Patient Responses**
   ◆ Compared with expected outcomes
   ◆ Compared with patient's baseline status

NURSING NOTES

The professional nurse uses all acquired skills in combination—**assessment, observation, intuition, diagnosis, planning, evaluation, documentation**—to provide the most effective nursing care for every patient.

Communication

Therapeutic Communication

- Relationships between patients and health care providers are based on trust and caring and cannot be achieved without a genuine concern for others.
- Therapeutic nurse/patient relationships can occur only when each person views the other as a unique human being.
- Therapeutic relationships are goal-directed and purposeful.
- Therapeutic interaction involves:
  - ◆ Establishing a contract for the time, place, and focus of the nurse/patient meetings.
  - ◆ Planning conditions for termination at the onset and ongoing throughout the relationship.
- Roles and responsibilities should be clearly defined:
  - ◆ The nurse is the professional caregiver and facilitator.
  - ◆ The patient's needs and problems are the focus of the relationship.
- Confidentiality is maintained by:
  - ◆ Sharing information only with professional staff who have a need to know.
  - ◆ Informing the patient of all information to be shared beforehand.
  - ◆ Advising the patient that information that deals with harming himself/herself or others will be communicated to the staff as needed.

Conditions Essential to a Therapeutic Relationship

Rapport	Implies special feelings on the part of both the patient and the nurse, based on acceptance, warmth, friendliness, common interest, a sense of trust and a nonjudgmental attitude.
Trust	Implies a feeling of confidence in another person's presence, reliability, integrity, veracity and sincere desire to provide assistance when requested; trust is the basis of a therapeutic relationship.
Respect	Implies the dignity and worth of an individual, regardless of his/her unacceptable behavior.
Genuineness	Refers to the nurse's ability to be open, honest and "real" in interactions with the patient; genuineness implies congruence between what is being felt and what is being expressed.
Empathy	A process wherein an individual is able to see beyond outward behavior and sense accurately another's inner experience at a given time; with empathy, the nurse's feelings remain on an objective level—it differs from sympathy in that, with sympathy, the nurse subjectively shares what the other person is feeling and experiences a personal need to alleviate distress.

Therapeutic Communication Techniques

Include verbal and nonverbal forms of communication:

■ **Silence:** Sitting quietly with a patient and nonverbally communicating interest and presence.

■ **Listening:** Maintaining eye contact and an open, receptive body position.

■ **Opening:** First comments to the patient—"What would you like to talk about today?" or "What brought you here today?"

■ **Restating:** Rephrasing the patient's words—"What I hear you saying is…" or "You said the doctors told you…"

■ **Clarification:** Helping the patient communicate more clearly—"Could you tell me again?" or "I'm not certain what you mean."

■ **Reflection:** Providing stability through communication—"You are feeling anxious and it is because you need to talk with the cardiologist."

■ **Focusing:** Helping the patient stay on topic—"Let's focus on your relationship with your son."

■ **Sharing Perceptions:** Offering observations without judgment—"You look upset, but are saying you are not bothered by the delay in your surgery?"

■ **Identifying Themes:** Helping the patient notice patterns of behavior or reaction—"I've noticed that in all the relationships you describe, you have been hurt by your partner. Do you think there is a theme?"

Barriers to Therapeutic Interactions

■ **Language Differences**

  ◆ Inability to communicate may affect the patient's response to interventions.

  ◆ Use of value-laden terms may block the exchange of information, ideas and feelings.

■ **Cultural Differences**

  ◆ Influence use of language.

  ◆ Depend upon variables such as eye contact, proximity to others, direct or indirect questions, role of informal conversation and decision-making patterns are influenced.

■ **Gender**

  ◆ Use of nonverbal cues are gender dependent.

  ◆ Women are more aware of nonverbal cues.

  ◆ Men prefer more personal distance between persons.

■ **Health Condition**

  ◆ Level of consciousness.

  ◆ Sensory perception alterations such as loss of vision or hearing.

■ **Developmental Level**

■ **Knowledge Differences**

■ **Emotions**

  ◆ Anxiety, fear and other emotions can change or interrupt the quality of communications.

■ **Use of Health-Care Jargon**

  ◆ Professional jargon may not be understood by the patient and, as a result, may become a block to effective communication.

Nonverbal Communication

■ Research suggests that nonverbal communication is more important in understanding human behavior than words alone—the nonverbal "channels" seem to be more powerful than what people say.

◆ **Eye Contact:** An important channel of interpersonal communication that helps regulate the flow of communication and also signals interest in others; furthermore, eye contact with patients increases the nurse's credibility, presence and dedication to others. Nurses who make eye contact open the flow of communication and convey interest, concern, warmth and trust.

◆ **Facial Expressions:** Smiling is a powerful cue that transmits happiness, friendliness, warmth, liking and affiliation; as a result, if you smile frequently, you will be perceived as more likable, friendly, warm and approachable; smiling is often contagious, and patients will react to it favorably.

◆ **Gestures:** Head nods, which are gestures, communicate positive reinforcement to patients and indicate that you are listening; if you fail to gesture while speaking, you may be perceived as boring, stiff and unanimated. A lively and animated style captures patients' attention, makes the material more interesting, facilitates learning and provides a bit of entertainment.

◆ **Posture & Body Orientation:** You communicate numerous messages by the way you walk, talk, stand and sit. Standing erect, but not rigid, and leaning slightly forward communicates to patients that you are approachable, receptive and friendly; furthermore, interpersonal closeness results when you and your patients face each other. Speaking with your back turned, and/or looking at the floor or ceiling, all should be avoided, as these positions communicate disinterest to your patients.

◆ **Proximity:** Cultural norms dictate a comfortable distance for interaction with patients. You should look for signals of discomfort caused by invading a patient's space, including rocking, leg swinging, tapping, gaze aversion.

◆ **Paralinguistics:** This facet of nonverbal communication includes such vocal elements as tone, pitch, rhythm, loudness and inflection.

NURSING NOTES

The professional nurse knows that communication is key to the patient's positive outcome. The nurse establishes **trust, respect, empathy, confidentiality** and **genuine caring** in every interaction with patients.

Comprehensive Health Assessment

■ A comprehensive health assessment includes all the dimensions of a person's health and also provides a baseline of the person's normal abilities, risk factors, and current description of health status.

■ The key to providing a thorough and effective nursing assessment is to ensure that a comprehensive health assessment is included.

■ Comprehensive health assessments encompass:

◆ **Physical Health:** Basic functions such as walking, eating and breathing.

◆ **Psychological Health:** Emotions and behaviors, including intellect and self-concept/self-image.

◆ **Social Health:** Relationships and interactions among persons.

◆ **Spiritual Health:** Belief in a higher being, attitudes toward moral decisions, and personal interpretation of the meaning of life.

Health History

A collection of data about the person's past and present functioning as related to his/her health.

■ **Components of a Health History**

◆ Biographical data

◆ Chief complaint: Patient's reason for seeking care. Use patient's own words.

◆ History of present illness

◆ **PQRST** mnemonic device
  • **P:** Provocation/Palliative: What causes it? What makes it better or worse?
  • **Q:** Quality/Quantity: How does it feel, look or sound, and how much of it is there?
  • **R:** Region/Radiation: Where is it? Does it spread?
  • **S:** Severity Scale: Does it interfere with activities of daily living?
  • **T:** Timing: When did it begin? How often does it occur? Is it gradual or sudden? How long does an episode of the symptom last?
◆ Past health history
  • Other health problems, allergies
  • Immunizations and childhood illnesses
  • Prior hospitalizations, pregnancy histories
◆ Current medications—prescription, OTC, vitamins and complementary therapies
◆ Family history
◆ Personal/social history
◆ Lifestyle assessment
  • Diet/nutrition
  • Activity and exercise
  • Sleep and rest
  • Tobacco, alcohol, drug use
  • Religion and spirituality
  • Social data
  • Living arrangements
  • Relationships (family and friends)
  • Psychological data
  • Occupation
  • Travel
  • Health resources

◆ Review of systems
  • This is a systematic review of the past and current health status of each body system.
  • Goal is to obtain subjective data or the patient's perception.

Techniques of Physical Assessment

Inspection

■ Observation of physical features and behaviors.
■ Use of all senses to gather data.
■ A purposeful and systematic comparison of bilateral body parts.

  ◆ **Concentrated Watching**
    • Scrutinize the individual as a whole.
    • Visually look at each system.
    • Compare right to left side using the person as their own control.

  ◆ **Active Listening**
    • Tone, pitch, pattern and speed of speech
    • Quality of vocalizations

  ◆ **Acute Smelling**
    • Odor assessment

Palpation

Touching with the hand and fingers to discriminate temperature, position, texture, size, consistency, masses and fluid.

■ **Superficial Palpation:** Feeling on the surface.

  ◆ Fingertips are used to differentiate fine differences in texture and consistency.
  ◆ Dorsum of hand is used to differentiate temperature.
  ◆ Palm of hand is used to locate vibrations.

■ **Light Palpation:** Using 3 to 4 fingers to depress an area of skin approximately 0.5–1 inch. Purpose is to detect masses and locate areas of discomfort.

■ **Deep Palpation:** Compressing an area to a depth of approximately 1.5–2 inches. Purpose is to locate organs, determine size and detect masses.

■ **Palpation of Edema:** Place thumb over edematous area (usually dorsum of foot or tibia) for 5 seconds and release.

◆ 0 : No edema
◆ 1+: barely visible depression
◆ 2+: depression less than 5 mm and normal contour of extremity
◆ 3+: depression of 5-10 mm and swelling of extremity.

■ **Palpation of Pulses:** Peripheral pulses are compared for rate, rhythm and quality.

◆ 0: absent
◆ +1: weak and thready
◆ +2: normal
◆ +3: full
◆ +4: bounding

■ **Palpation of Muscle Strength**

◆ Muscle Strength Assessment

5	Normal strength. Muscle is able to move through a full range of motion (ROM) against gravity and applied resistance.
4	Muscle is able to move through a full ROM against gravity but with weakness to applied resistance.
3	Muscle is able to move alone actively against gravity.
2	Muscle is able to move with support against gravity.

1	Muscle contraction is palpable and visible.
0	Muscle contraction or movement is undetectable.

Percussion

Producing resonance (sound) by striking one object against another to determine density of underlying structures.

■ **Direct Percussion:** Tapping an area directly with the tips of the middle fingers.

■ **Indirect Percussion:** Placing the non-dominant hand's fingers on the area to be percussed and using the dominant hand to strike those fingers and produce a sound.

◆ **Characteristics of Percussion Sounds**

- **Tympany:** Loud, drum-like sound.
  > Location: Air-filled stomach, intestines.
- **Hyperresonance:** Very loud, very low-pitched booming sound.
  > Location: Emphysematous lung.
- **Resonance:** Loud, low-pitched, hollow sound.
  > Location: Normal lung.
- **Dullness:** Medium intensity and pitch, thud-like.
  > Location: Liver or diaphragm.
- **Flatness:** Soft and high-pitched.
  > Location: Muscle or bone.

Auscultation

Listening for sounds of movement within the body, such as movement of blood in the heart and vessels, and movement of air in the lungs and intestines.

■ **Heart Sounds:** Produced by valve closure. Heard where blood flows away from the valve, not directly over the valve.

◆ **Normal Heart Sounds**
- **S1:** Beginning of systolic phase or the closure of the mitral and tricuspid (AV) valves; simultaneous with carotid pulse.
- **S2:** Beginning of diastolic phase or the closure of the aortic and pulmonic valve.

◆ Abnormal Heart Sounds
- **S3:** Ventricle filling sound occurs early in diastole.
- **S4:** Atrial contraction occurs later in diastole.
- **Murmur:** Turbulent or obstructed blood flow resulting in vibrating sound.

■ **Lung Sounds:** Produced by movement of air with each inspiration and expiration.

◆ **Normal Breath Sounds**
- **Vesicular breath sounds:** Soft, breezy, low-pitched sound that is heard over all peripheral lung fields, especially in the bases. Inspiration phase is longer than expiration.
- **Bronchovesicular:** Breezy, soft and lower pitched than bronchial sounds. Heard from the anterior at bifurcation of main bronchi and from the posterior between the scapulas. Inspiratory phase is equal to expiratory phase.
- **Bronchial breath sounds:** Hollow, loud, high-pitched sound. Heard over trachea. Expiratory phase is longer than inspiration.

◆ **Adventitious Breath Sounds:** Abnormal sound of air passing through narrowed airways or through fluid-filled or inflamed tissue.
- **Crackles:** Air passing though fluid or exudates.
  > **Sound:** Crackling, popping, moist, bubbling sound heard on inspiration, primarily in the

alveoli and peripheral airways. Unrelieved by coughing.

> **Associated conditions:** Restrictive diseases such as pneumonia, congestive heart failure, pulmonary edema and pulmonary fibrosis.

- **Gurgles/Rhonchi/Wheezes (Sonorous):** Air passing through airways constricted as a result of swelling, secretion or tumor.

  > **Sound:** Rumbling, snoring or moaning sound heard on expiration, primarily in the large airways. Relieved by coughing.

  > **Associated conditions:** Bronchitis or single bronchus obstruction, pneumonia.

- **Wheezes (Sibilant):** Air passing through airways constricted as a result of swelling, secretion or tumor.

  > **Sound:** High-pitched musical sound, heard primarily on expiration, but may be heard on inspiration. Found in both large and small airways.

  > **Associated conditions:** Acute asthma and chronic emphysema.

- **Stridor:** Air movement through progressive narrowing of upper airway.

  > **Sound:** Harsh, high-pitched, heard on inspiration and expiration. In severe cases, audible without stethoscope.

  > **Associated conditions:** Partial airway obstruction, croup, epiglottitis.

- **Pleural Friction Rub:** Rubbing of inflamed pleural surfaces.

  > **Sound:** Dry, grating sound heard on both inspiration and expiration.

  > **Associated conditions:** Pleuritis.

- **Bronchophony:** Ask patient to repeat "ninety-nine." If the auscultated sound is loud and clear it indicates consolidation or atelectasis.
- **Egophony:** Ask patient to repeat "ee." If the auscultated sound is "ay" it indicates consolidation or atelectasis.

◆ **Bowel Sounds**
  - Normal: Every 15 to 20 seconds.
  - Hypoactive: Every 60 seconds or more.
  - Hyperactive: Every 3 seconds (approximately).

■ A **stethoscope** is used to collect and transmit sounds.

  ◆ **Diaphragm:** Pressed firmly to the skin to detect high pitched sound, i.e. breath sounds, heart sound, bowel sounds.
  ◆ **Belly:** Placed lightly on the skin to detect low-pitched sounds (i.e., abnormal heart sound, bruits).

Basic Head-to-Toe Assessment

Area Assessed	Assessment Technique	Assessment Parameters
General Survey	Inspect	• Overall appearance of health • Signs of distress • Expression and mood • Level of consciousness and cognition • Body size, grooming and hygiene • Skin: condition, color, temperature, presence of lesions, injury, odor • Vital signs and weight

Area Assessed	Assessment Technique	Assessment Parameters
Head	Inspect and palpate	• Skull size, shape, symmetry, condition of hair and scalp • Facial symmetry
Eyes	Inspect	• Color and hydration of conjunctiva • PERRLA: Pupils equal, round, reactive to light and accommodation • EOM: Extra-ocular movements • Ophthalmoscope examination of retina
Ears	Inspect	• Hearing acuity • Rinne and Weber test • Visualize tympanic membrane with otoscope
Nose	Inspect	• Congestion, drainage, sense of smell • Patency of nares, septal deviation • Nasal flaring
Mouth & Throat	Inspect	• Condition of mucous membrane, teeth, tongue, oropharynx

Area Assessed	Assessment Technique	Assessment Parameters
Mouth & Throat *(cont.)*	Inspect	• Clench jaw, puff out cheeks with air • Gag reflex, rise of uvula
	Palpate	• Temporomandibular joint movement
Neck	Inspect	• Range of motion, stiffness or pain • Symmetry • Jugular vein distension
	Palpate	• Jugular vein distension, tracheal alignment, muscle strength • Carotid pulses • Cervical lymph nodes • Thyroid gland
	Auscultate	• Bruits
Upper Extremities	Inspect	• Skin: color, temperature, condition • Nails: blanche for capillary refill, clubbing • Presence of edema • Range of motion

Area Assessed	Assessment Technique	Assessment Parameters
Upper Extremities *(cont.)*	Palpate	• Peripheral pulses (radial): strength, rate, symmetry • Muscle strength and resistance
	Percuss	• Deep tendon reflexes
Posterior Thorax	Inspect	• Spinal alignment • Anterior-posterior to lateral diameter of thorax • Thoracic expansion
	Palpate	• Tactile fremetus
	Auscultate	• Breath sounds
Anterior Thorax	Inspect	• Inspect condition and appearance of skin, presence of scars, symmetry and shape of chest, movement, deformity, point of maximal impulse (PMI or apical pulse) • Respiratory pattern: depth, pattern, effort—use of accessory muscles

Area Assessed	Assessment Technique	Assessment Parameters
Anterior Thorax *(cont.)*	Palpate	• PMI for lifts, thrills, vibrations or heaves • Respiratory excursion • Breast examination
	Auscultate	• Breath sounds • Heart sounds
Abdomen	Inspect	• Skin distension, scars, obesity, herniations, bruising, pulsations
	Auscultate	• Bowel sounds
	Percuss	• Location and size of organs (liver, spleen)
	Palpate	• Pulsations, masses, tenderness, rigidity • Palpate kidney
Lower Extremities	Inspect	• Skin: condition, color, temperature • Edema • Range of motion
	Palpate	• Peripheral pulses (dorsal pedis, posterior tibial) • Edema • Homan's sign • Joints for swelling

Area Assessed	Assessment Technique	Assessment Parameters
Neurological	Inspect	• Temperature, sensory perception • Gait and balance • Recent and remote memory • Cerebellar function: finger to nose test, heel to shin • Two point discrimination

NURSING NOTES

The professional nurse recognizes the importance of the **comprehensive health assessment**, paying equal attention to obtaining the patient's **health history** and providing a **basic head-to-toe physical assessment** (using *inspection, palpation, percussion, auscultation*).

Patient Education

Teaching/Learning

A planned interactional process that promotes intentional behavioral change.

Purposes of Patient Teaching

- ■ Promotion of wellness
- ■ Prevention of disease/injury
- ■ Restoration of health
- ■ Facilitation of coping abilities
- ■ Providing education in a manner that:
  - ◆ Facilitates understanding of the patient's health status, health-care options, and the health-care options selected.
  - ◆ Encourages participation in decision making about health-care options.
  - ◆ Increases the potential for patient and/or significant other to follow the therapeutic health-care options.
  - ◆ Maximizes care skills.
  - ◆ Increases the ability of the patient and/or significant other to cope with the patient's health status, prognosis, outcome.
  - ◆ Enhances the patient's and/or significant other's role and understanding of their responsibility in continuing care and promoting a healthy lifestyle.

Domains of Learning

■ **Cognitive:** Rational thought or thinking.
  ◆ Learning facts, reaching conclusions, solving problems, making decisions and using critical thinking skills.
    • Example: Patient can state the name and purpose of his/her medicines.
■ **Affective:** Emotions or feelings.
  ◆ Changing beliefs, attitudes or values used in making judgments.
  ◆ Difficult to measure because it focuses on thoughts and feelings.
    • Example: Patient accepts that he/she has a chronic illness.
■ **Psychomotor:** Physical application of knowledge.
  ◆ Muscular movements learned to perform a new skill or procedure.
  ◆ Easiest to measure because it can be physically demonstrated.
    • Example: Patient demonstrates self-catheterization.

Planning for Teaching/Learning Encounters

■ Focus on the patient.
■ Consider the whole person, not just specific content.
■ **Baseline Knowledge:** Previous patient education experiences and existing knowledge. Determine what is known and build from there.
■ **Cultural & Language Needs:** Consider components of diversity such as race/ethnicity, religion, health beliefs, language, and sex-role beliefs.

- **Priorities:** Determine the patient's learning needs.
- **Realistic Approach:** Consider the patient's age, energy level and emotional state.

Key Points for a Teaching Session
- Focus on patient's perspective.
- Emphasize what to do and why, not what to know.
- Keep it simple.
- Provide small, vital bits of information, one at a time.
- Focus on main objectives.
- Use short sentences, concrete language, but not jargon.
- Repeat the main topic point at the end as a summary.
- Ask patient to re-state what you said.
- Use printed material to highlight specific phases.
- Give educational materials that promote active involvement.
- Use positive words, phrases and messages; avoid scare tactics.
- Evaluate ongoing.

Learning Opportunities in Health Care
- Find the "teachable moment" and seize it.
- Make sure that the patient's basic physiological needs are met.
- He/she is comfortable.
- He/she is ready to learn.

Opportunity

Admission

Beginning of Each Shift

New Medications

Diagnostic Procedure

Surgery

Discharge

Teaching/Learning Across the Life Span

- All people are capable of learning.
- Learning needs and abilities are influenced by chronological and developmental age.
- Teaching strategies need to be modified for different age groups.

Age	Developmental Teaching Needs
Infant Learn through interaction with their environment.	• Immunizations • Growth/development concepts • Infant safety • Nutrition • Sleep patterns • Skin integrity • Sensory stimulation

Learning Needs

•Coming to know a new environment.
•Understanding specific treatment and their purpose.

•Explaining new treatment or changes in plan of care.
•Assessing patient's need to know.

•Knowing action of drug, dosage, side effects.
•Demonstrating proper use and storage.

•Knowing necessary preparation and what will happen.

•Explaining pre-operative routine and preparations.
•Practicing protocols such as leg exercises, coughing
and deep breathing, log rolling, or getting out of bed,
in preparation for post-operative period.

•Knowing any limitations on daily activities.
•Demonstrating ability to care for self.

NURSING NOTES

The professional nurse is aware of the
importance of patient education and assists the
patient's learning (in a manner appropriate to
patient's age, development and abilities) in order
to achieve optimal effectiveness of nursing care.

Teaching Strategies

- Be consistent
- Use brightly colored
  toys, objects
- Role model nurturing
  role for parent

Nursing Considerations

- Teach to primary caregiver.
- Emphasize need for
  consistency.
- Encourage an environment
  rich in appropriate stimuli
  to promote cognitive
  development.

Age	Developmental Teaching Needs
Toddler Parents are the most effective teachers – involve them.	• Accident prevention • Toilet training • Dental care • Play activities • Immunizations • Nutrition
Preschool Trust is vital. They like to be proud of their accomplishments.	• Accident prevention • Dental health • Nutrition • Cognitive stimulation • Sleep patterns
School Age Usually eager to learn and understand cause and effect.	• Dental hygiene • Safety measures • Physical activity and fitness • Hygiene • Socialization with peers
Adolescent Appreciate open, honest and complete answers to their questions. Maintain confidentiality.	• Effects of drugs and alcohol • Safe sexual behaviors • Sexually transmitted infections • Reducing risk of injury • Nutrition • Changing body shape and size

Teaching Strategies	Nursing Considerations
• Play with appropriate equipment • Positive simple commands • Picture books • Puppets, dolls	• Involve parent to decrease anxiety. • Assess for sensory overload. • Don't try to teach.
• Immediate reinforcement for positive behaviors • Play • Music, singing movement	• Often uses words without knowing the meaning. • Feelings are expressed through actions, not words.
• Toys • Game and books • Demonstration • Role playing	• Can follow simple directions. • Include them in planning and goal setting. • Seeks approval for doing the right thing. • Assess ability to read.
• Printed material appropriate to age/literacy level • Role playing • Demonstration • Peer support	• Maintain privacy. • Assess for and correct misinformation. • A sense of invulnerability can lead to a "not me" attitude. • Emphasize immediate benefit of learning information.

Age	Developmental Teaching Needs	Teaching Strategies	Nursing Considerations
Young/Middle-Aged Adult Motivated by activities that enhance self-esteem. Middle adults do not take good health for granted.	• Importance of preventative health screenings • Sun protection • Nutrition • Exercise • Stress/time management • Parenting skills	• Printed materials appropriate to literacy level • Discussion • Demonstration • Role playing	• Encourage input and mutual planning/goal setting. • Increased awareness of vulnerability with age.
Older Adult Physiological changes of aging may hinder learning.	• Exercise to maintain mobility • Nutritional information • Fall prevention • Loss and grief • Stress management • Socialization	• Assess for reading/hearing skills • Repeat frequently • Demonstration • Discussion	• Show strong desire for independence. • Aging does not lead to decreased intelligence.

5 Basic Patient Needs & Nursing Care

■ Physiological needs of the patient enable homeostasis and are the highest priority.

■ When a physiological need is unmet, it can control a patient's thoughts and behavior and can cause the person to feel sickness, pain and discomfort.

Vital Signs (VS)

■ Vital signs **(VS)** are physical signs that indicate an individual is alive, such as heartbeat, breathing rate, temperature, and blood pressure. These signs can be observed, measured, and monitored to assess an individual's level of physical functioning.

■ Normal VS can change with age, sex, weight, exercise tolerance, and condition.

■ These numbers provide critical information (hence the name "**vital**") about a patient's state of health.

■ In particular, they:
- ◆ Can identify the existence of an acute medical problem.
- ◆ Are a means of rapidly quantifying the magnitude of an illness and how well the body is coping with the resultant physiological stress. The more deranged the vitals, the sicker the patient.
- ◆ Are markers of chronic disease states (e.g., hypertension is defined as chronically elevated blood pressure).

Getting Started

■ The examination/hospital room should be quiet, warm and well lit.

■ Prior to measuring vital signs, the patient should have the opportunity to sit or rest in bed for approximately five minutes so that the values are not affected by the exertion required to walk to the exam room or other activities.

■ All measurements are made while the patient is sitting/reclining.

Observation

■ Before diving in, take a minute or so to look at the patient in his/her entirety, making your observations, if possible, from an out-of-the way perch. Does the patient seem anxious, in pain, upset? What about their dress and hygiene?

■ Remember, the data collection process begins as soon as you lay eyes on the patient.

Temperature
■ **Normal = 98.6° F**

■ Obtained using an oral thermometer that provides a digital reading when the sensor is placed under the patient's tongue.

■ Temperature is measured in degrees, either Celsius (C) or Fahrenheit (F).

■ Rectal temperature, which most closely reflects internal or core temperature, is approximately one degree Fahrenheit (1° F) higher than those obtained orally.

■ A **fever** is defined as greater than 38–38.5° C or 101–101.5° F.

Respiratory Rate
■ **12 to 18 respirations (breaths) per minute**

- Respirations should be counted for at least 30 seconds. The total number of breaths in a 15 second period is relatively small, and any miscounting can result in rather large errors when multiplied by 4.
- Try to count respirations as surreptitiously as possible so that the patient does not consciously alter his/her rate of breathing. This can be done by observing the rise and fall of the patient's hospital gown while you appear to be taking his/her pulse.
- Respiratory rate, particularly in the presence of cardiopulmonary illness, can be a very reliable marker of disease activity.

Pulse

- **60 to 80 beats per minute (at rest)**
- Can be measured at any place where there is a large artery (e.g., carotid or femoral) or simply by listening over the heart.
- For the sake of convenience, it is generally done by palpating the radial impulse: Place the tips of your index and middle fingers just proximal to the patient's wrist on the thumb side, orienting them so that they both are over the length of the vessel.

Blood Pressure (BP)

- **Systolic: less than 120 mm of mercury (mm Hg)**
- **Diastolic: less than 80 mm Hg**
- Readings are reported in millimeters of mercury **(mm Hg).**
- The size of the BP cuff will affect the accuracy of these readings.
  - ◆ The inflatable bladder, which can be felt through the vinyl covering of the cuff, should reach approximately 80% around the circumference of the arm.

◆ The width of the inflatable bladder should cover approximately 40%. If the cuff is too small, the readings will be artificially elevated. If the cuff is too large, the readings will be artificially low.

> ## NURSING NOTES
> Vital signs are VITAL!
> The professional nurse takes care to ensure the **accuracy** of vital signs, as well as the **patient's comfort** while obtaining them.

Fluid Balance & Imbalance

The body normally maintains a balance between the amount of fluid taken in and the amount of fluid excreted.

■ The body's fluid is contained within 3 compartments:
- ◆ **Intracellular:** within the cell
- ◆ **Intravascular:** within blood vessels
- ◆ **Interstitial:** between cells

■ There are 2 types of body fluids:
- ◆ **Intracellular Fluid (ICF):** fluid within the cells; most stable component
- ◆ **Extracellular Fluid (ECF):** fluid outside the cells
- ◆ **Intravascular Fluid:** within the blood vessels; least stable
- ◆ **Interstitial Fluid:** fluid surrounding the cells; reserve fluid

■ **Water** is the largest component of the body's fluids.

■ About $2/3$ of the body's fluid is intracellular.

■ The remaining $1/3$ is extracellular.

■ About 25% is intravascular while 75% is interstitial.

■ Water is present in all body tissues and cells.

Electrolytes

- Compounds that, when dissolved in water, form or dissociate into ions.
- Electrolytes provide inorganic chemicals for cellular reactions and control mechanisms.
- Electrolytes have special physiological functions in the body that:
  - ◆ Promote neuromuscular irritability.
  - ◆ Maintain body fluid's osmolarity.
  - ◆ Regulate acid/base balance.
  - ◆ Distribute body fluids between the fluid compartments.

Regulators of Fluid Balance

- Fluid and food intake and loss.
- Water enters the body as:
  - ◆ Oral liquids
  - ◆ Water in foods
  - ◆ Waste formed by oxidation of foods

Ingested liquids	1,500 ml
Water in foods	700 ml
Water from oxidation	200 ml
Total Normal Daily Fluid Intake (adult)	2,400 ml

- **Skin:** Diffusion through the skin results in an estimated water loss of 300 to 400 ml per day. This is referred to as **ISWL (insensible water loss)**. A common form of ISWL is perspiration.
- **Lungs:** Expired air is saturated with water vapor resulting in additional ISWL.

■ **Gastrointestinal (GI) Tract:** Most of the fluid secreted into the GI tract is reabsorbed by the body—about 200 ml per day is lost in fecal material.

■ **Kidneys:** Excrete 1,200–1,500 ml/day in the adult. The excretion of water by the healthy kidney is proportional to the fluid ingested and the amount of waste and solutes excreted. The interaction of renal hormones serves as the body's compensatory mechanism to maintain homeostasis.

  ♦ **ADH (antidiuretic hormone)** from the posterior pituitary gland acts on the distal tubules of the kidneys to reabsorb water.

  ♦ **Aldosterone** causes the reabsorption of sodium from the renal tubules, leading to water retention and increased extracellular volume.

  ♦ **Renin** promotes vasoconstriction and the release of aldosterone.

Disturbances in Electrolyte & Acid/Base Balance

Normal homeostatic mechanisms function to maintain electrolytes and acid/base balance.

■ **Sodium:** The primary determinant of extracellular fluid concentration because of its high concentration and inability to cross the cell membrane easily.

  ♦ Alterations in sodium concentration can result in profound CNS effects on cognition and sensory perception and on circulating blood volume.

    • **Hyponatremia:** Deficit in extracellular sodium level due to water deficit or water excess. A hypo-osmolar state (water concentration greater than sodium concentration) results in water moving out of the vascular space into the interstitial space and then into the intracellular space, causing edema (e.g., cerebral edema).

- **Hypernatremia:** Excess of sodium in the extracellular fluid. Hyper-osmolar state (sodium concentration greater than water concentration) causes an increase in the extracellular osmotic pressure, pulling fluid out of the cells and into the extracellular space.

■ **Potassium:** The normal range of extracellular potassium (K+) is narrow (3.5–5.0 mEq/L). Potassium has a vital role in cardiac muscle contraction and, therefore, monitoring and maintaining a normal concentration is vital.

- ◆ A reciprocal relationship exists between sodium and potassium: a large sodium intake results in an increased loss of potassium and vice versa.
  - **Hypokalemia:** Decrease in the extracellular level of potassium. GI tract disturbances (e.g., vomiting or diarrhea) and the use of diuretics place the patient at risk for hypokalemia.
  - **Hyperkalemia:** Increased extracellular level of potassium.

Potassium Chloride (KCl)

NEVER administer more than 10 mEq of intravenous KCl per hour.

The normal dose of intravenous KCl is 20–40 mEq to infuse over an 8-hour period.

Nursing Assessment

Assessment data is collected to identify patients who have potential or actual alterations in fluid volume.

■ **Health History:** Elicit data specific to fluids.
  - ◆ Dietary intake

◆ Weight – usual patterns and recent changes
◆ Fluid output – usual patterns (urinary and bowel) and recent changes
◆ GI disturbances
◆ Fever and diaphoresis
◆ Draining wounds, burns or trauma

Physical Examination

■ Daily Weight

◆ Change in total body fluid volume is reflected in weight.
◆ A kilogram (2.2 lbs) of body weight (sudden gain or loss) is equivalent to one liter (1,000 ml) of fluid gained or lost.
◆ Accurate measurement of daily weight (same time, same scale, same clothing) reveals changes in fluid volume.

■ Vital Signs (VS)

◆ An elevated temperature may indicate dehydration and places the patient at risk for dehydration because of increased loss of body fluids.
◆ Changes in pulse rate and characteristics reflect fluid volume.
◆ Respiratory changes (in depth or rate) may indicate acid/base imbalances. Also, increased respiratory rate leads to increased ISWL.
◆ **BP:** assess fluid volume. A narrowed pulse pressure may indicate a fluid volume deficit.

■ Intake & Output

◆ Measurement for a 24-hour period identifies potential or actual imbalances.
◆ A minimum intake of 1,500 ml is essential to balance urinary output and the body's ISWL.

◆ Intake includes all liquids (food substances that are liquid at room temperature) taken by mouth and liquids administered through tubes and parenterally.

◆ Output includes urine, diarrhea, vomitus, and drainage from tubes.

■ **Edema**

◆ The detectable accumulation of increased interstitial fluid.

◆ Edema may be localized or generalized.

◆ Localized edema is characterized by taut, smooth, shiny, pale skin—often found in dependent post parts.

■ **Skin Turgor:** The normal resiliency of the skin.

■ **Buccal (Oral) Cavity:** Inspect the oral mucous membranes: decreased saliva, dry membranes and cracked lips are signs of fluid volume deficit.

■ **Eyes:** Sunken, dry eyes (absence of tearing) are signs of fluid deficit, whereas puffy eyelids (papilledema) characterize fluid excess.

■ **Jugular Veins:** Measuring venous filling of the jugular and hand veins.

Nursing Care Responsibilities

Nursing care related to alterations in body fluid or electrolytes is based on the goal of maintaining homeostasis, and regulating and maintaining essential fluids and nutrients. The nurse's responsibilities include the need to:

■ Understand the patient's metabolic needs and make judgments concerning the outcome of therapy.

■ Perform frequent assessment and monitoring to recognize the adverse effects of fluid and electrolytes therapy and to prevent complications.

■ Prevent the rapid depletion of the body's protein and energy reserves.

■ **Monitor Daily Weight:** A main indicator of water and electrolyte balance.
  ◆ Weight is obtained every day in the AM, at the same time, using the same scale, and with the patient dressed in the same type of clothing.

■ **Measure Vital Signs (VS):** VS in conjunction with other clinical data are used to determine the type and amount of fluid therapy.

■ **Measure Intake & Output (I & O):** Evaluate the patient's fluid status over a 24-hour period.
  ◆ Strict I & O requires accounting for incontinent urine, emesis, and diaphoresis, and requires weighing soiled bed linen, gown and other items.
  ◆ A patient's intake should exceed output by 500 ml to account for ISWL. I & O and daily weights are critical intervention because they not only measure current fluid status but also the effectiveness of diuretic or rehydration therapy.
  ◆ Obtaining an accurate I & O requires the support of the patient and family.

■ **Provide Oral Hygiene:** Oral care promotes comfort and integrity of the buccal mucosa.
  ◆ A dehydrated patient has decreased saliva production and is at risk for development of oral lesions or disease.
  ◆ Avoid overuse of mouthwash or glycerin swabs, which contain alcohol. While these items initially feel refreshing, they have a drying effect on the mucous membranes.

■ **Initiate Oral Fluid Therapy:** Oral fluids my be totally restricted, limited or forced, depending on the patient's clinical situation.

◆ **NPO (*Non per os* – nothing by mouth):** Patient needs frequent mouth hygiene (q 1–2 hours) for comfort and to prevent mouth ulcers. Used in situations that include the need to:
  • Avoid aspiration in unconscious, perioperative and pre-procedural patients who will receive anesthesia or conscious sedation.
  • Rest and heal the GI tract in patients with severe vomiting or diarrhea, or when the patient has a GI disorder (inflammation or obstruction).
  • Prevent the further loss of gastric juices in patients with nasogastric suctioning.
◆ **Restricted Fluids:** Intake may be restricted to as little as 200 ml over a 24-hour period.
  • Fluid restriction is commonly used in the treatment of excessive fluid volume related to heart and renal failure.
  • How fluids will be restricted should be determined in collaboration with the patient, for example:
    > 50% of allowed fluids are taken at breakfast and lunch.
    > Remaining 50% might be taken with the evening meal and HS (bedtime) snack.
◆ **Forced Fluids:** Encouraging fluid intake, especially water, may be done for patients at risk for dehydration or patients with renal and urinary problems.
  • A patient might be requested to consume 2,000 ml of fluid over 24 hours.
  • The largest quantity of fluid should be given with meals.

- *Remember that fluids include substances that are liquid at room temperature such as ice, gelatin and ice cream.*

■ **Maintain Tube Feedings:** Tube feedings as prescribed by the provider are used when the patient is unable to ingest oral fluids but has a normal GI tract.

■ **Monitor Intravenous Therapy:** Intravenous (IV) therapy (or parenteral fluid therapy) is the administration of fluids, electrolytes, nutrients or medication by the venous route.

NURSING NOTES

Balancing fluids is essential to the patient's therapy, as well as to the ongoing maintenance of health and well-being. The professional nurse ensures **effective fluid balance** and educates the patient on maintaining it as part of ongoing lifestyle modifications.

Elimination

■ The urinary and the gastrointestinal (GI) systems provide for the elimination of body waste.

■ Elimination patterns are essential to maintaining health and well-being.

■ The urinary system filters and excretes urine from the body and maintains fluid, electrolyte and acid/base balance.

■ Normal GI (bowel) function provides for the regular elimination of solid wastes.

■ Elimination patterns may be altered during periods of stress and illness.

■ Nurses play an active role in assisting the patient

with maintaining proper elimination patterns through assessment for changes, identification of problems, and interventions to promote effective elimination of bodily wastes.

Physiology of Urinary Elimination

■ The physiological process of urinary elimination is complex.

■ Continence requires anatomic integrity of the urinary system, nervous control of the detrusor muscle, and a competent sphincter mechanism.

■ The **upper urinary tract** includes:

◆ **The kidneys:** A pair of bean-shaped organs in the retroperitoneal space.

◆ **The renal pelvis:** A funnel-shaped reservoir that holds approximately 15 ml of urine.

◆ **The ureter:** A long tube shaped like an inverted "S."

■ The **lower urinary tract** includes:

◆ **The bladder:** A muscular organ in the pelvis with a fixed base and a distensile upper portion.

◆ **The urethra:** A tube that is the conduit for urinary elimination.

◆ **The pelvic muscle:** Connect the anterior and posterior aspects of the bony pelvis, support the organs of the true pelvis, and contribute to the urethral sphincter mechanism.

◆ The lower urinary tract, specifically the urethra, is *significantly different* in males and females.

Physiology of Bowel Elimination

■ Fecal continence primarily relies on the consistency of the stool (fecal material), intestinal motility, compliance and contractility of the rectum, and competence of the anal sphincter.

■ The GI tract begins at the mouth and ends at the anus.

■ The **upper GI tract** is primarily responsible for the ingestion, processing and preliminary digestion of foods.

■ The **lower GI tract** is primarily responsible for the latter stages of digestion, absorption and elimination.

◆ The **small intestine** is primarily responsible for the digestion and absorption of nutrients, vitamins, minerals, fluids and electrolytes.

◆ The **colon (large intestine)** is about 5 to 6 feet in length and its primary function is to collect, concentrate, transport and eliminate waste materials or feces.

◆ The **anal sphincter** consists of smooth and skeletal muscles that line the distal portion of the anal canal and works with the anus to store and eliminate feces under voluntary control.

◆ The transit time from ingestion of food to passage of stool varies. Transit time is significantly affected by the type of food ingested, exercise and stress-related factors.

Factors Affecting Elimination

■ **Age:** Age and/or developmental level affect control over urinary and bowel habits.

■ **Diet:** Adequate fluid and fiber intake are factors critical to maintaining urinary and bowel health.

◆ **Diarrhea** and **flatulence** (discharge of gas from the rectum) are a direct result of foods ingested.

■ **Exercise:** Enhances muscle tone and leads to better sphincter control.

◆ **Peristalsis** is also aided by activity.

■ **Medications:** Can have an impact on elimination health and patterns:

- ◆ **Diuretics** used by cardiac patients increase urine production.
- ◆ **OTC (over the counter) cold remedies**—especially antihistamines—may result in urine retention.
- ◆ **OTC laxatives** or stool softeners promote bowel elimination.
- ◆ **Codeine** may slow GI motility and lead to constipation.

Common Alterations in Elimination

- ■ The *most common alterations* in **urinary** elimination are **incontinence** (uncontrollable loss of urine) and **retention** (inability to completely empty the bladder).
- ■ The *primary alterations* in bowel elimination are:
  - ◆ **Constipation:** The infrequent and difficult passage of hardened stool.
  - ◆ **Diarrhea:** The passage of liquefied stool.
  - ◆ **Fecal Incontinence:** The involuntary loss of stool of sufficient magnitude to create a social and/or hygienic problem.

Nursing Care Responsibilities

All patients need to be taught basic principles of maintaining urinary and bowel elimination patterns.

- ■ **Fluid Intake:** The recommended daily allowance for fluids is 30 ml/kg of body weight. For the average-sized adult, this is **1,500 to 2,000 ml/day.**
- ■ **Diet:** Dietary fiber (fiber-rich food such as grains, fruits and vegetables) may prevent constipation.
- ■ Some foods and beverages are **bladder irritants**:
  - ◆ Caffeinated beverages, carbonated drinks and acidic fluids (coffee and tea)
  - ◆ Aspartame
  - ◆ Citrus fruits or juices

- ◆ Foods containing tomatoes or tomato-based sauces
- ◆ Chocolate
- ◆ Greasy or spicy foods

■ **Lifestyle & Prevention:** A healthy lifestyle can lead to healthy elimination patterns.

- ◆ **Alcohol:** Antidiuretic hormone (ADH) excreted by the hypothalamus is suppressed by alcohol intake, leading to **polyuria** (excess urine production). Alcohol also irritates the intestines and bowel, causing inflammation that results in **diarrhea.**

- ◆ **Tobacco:** Smoking increases the risk of **stress incontinence** because of its association with chronic coughing. Smoking also increases the risk for the development of **bladder cancer**. Smoking can stimulate the bowel, resulting in **diarrhea**.

- ◆ **Elimination Habits:** Individuals should establish regular patterns of elimination and answer the desire to defecate.

  - • **Positioning:** Sitting is the usual position for defecation. Women sit to urinate whereas men prefer to stand. Therefore, when using a bedpan, the head of the bed needs to be elevated as much as possible (unless contraindicated by medical condition).

  - • **Exercise regimen:** Exercise leads to good muscle tone and body metabolism, which stimulates the elimination in both the bowel and urinary systems.

  - • **Environmental modifications:** Remove environmental barriers, avoid difficult-to-manipulate clothing, and alter seating and toilets to enhance accessibility. Most important—**provide PRIVACY**.

NURSING NOTES
As stated above, *privacy is key*. The professional nurse blends **clinical knowledge** with **respect** and **empathy** to assist the patient's elimination functions.

Oxygenation

- Oxygenation, the delivery of oxygen (O_2) to the body's tissues and cells, is necessary to maintain life and health.
- When a patient's O_2 status is altered or compromised, careful assessment and thorough nursing care is essential to restore an effective and comfortable level of oxygenation function.

Physiology of Oxygenation

The delivery of O_2 to the body's cells involves the interplay of the **pulmonary, hematologic** and **cardiovascular** systems in 4 specific processes:

- Ventilation
- Diffusion (alveolar gas exchange)
- Perfusion (O_2 transport and delivery)
- Cellular respiration

Ventilation

- The movement of air into and out of the lungs for the purpose of delivering fresh air.
- Ventilation is regulated by respiratory control centers in the pons and medulla oblongata, located in the brain stem.
- The rate and depth of ventilation are constantly adjusted in response to changes in the concentration of hydrogen ions (pH) and carbon dioxide (CO_2) in the body fluids.

■ The mechanics of spontaneous ventilation is initiated when the diaphragm contracts, pulling it downward and thereby increasing the size of the intrathoracic space.

■ Concurrently, there is expansion/contraction of the external intercostal muscles, which elevate and separate the ribs and move the sternum forward. The additive effect of increasing the intrathoracic space is to decrease intrathoracic pressure and to draw air in from the atmosphere.

◆ This is the process of **inhalation**. When the lungs are filled with air, stretch receptors send signals to the brain to cease the process of inhalation.

◆ **Exhalation,** a passive process, occurs as the respiratory muscles relax, thereby reducing the size of the intrathoracic space, increasing the intrathoracic pressure and forcing air to exit the lungs.

◆ This entire muscular process is referred to as the work of **breathing**.

◆ The work of breathing is increased when the movement of air is impeded and additional muscles (known as accessory muscles) are used for the ventilatory process. These accessory muscles include the **sternocleidomastoid** muscle, the **abdominal** muscles and the **internal intercostal** muscles.

Diffusion (Alveolar Gas Exchange)

■ The exchange of O_2 from the alveolar space into the pulmonary capillary blood is called **oxygen uptake.**

◆ **O_2 diffuses** across the **alveolar membrane** in response to a concentration gradient; in other words, it moves from an area of higher concentration (the alveoli) to an area of lower concentration (pulmonary capillary blood), seeking *concentration equilibrium.*

Perfusion (O_2 Transport & Delivery)

■ The process of O_2 molecules *dissolving* into the blood plasma and oxygenation tissue and organs is **perfusion**.

■ 3 factors influence the capacity of the blood to carry O_2:

  ◆ The amount of dissolved O_2 in the plasma.

  ◆ The amount of hemoglobin.

  ◆ The tendency of the hemoglobin to bind with O_2.

■ Because O_2 is bound to hemoglobin, the O_2's delivery to the body's cells is accomplished through the process of **circulation.**

■ Circulation of the blood is the function of the heart and blood vessels.

■ The heart is the muscular pump of the circulatory process. A single cycle of **contraction** of the heart's chambers (atria and ventricles) and **relaxation** is called the cardiac cycle.

■ Basically the cardiac cycle consist of 2 processes:

  ◆ **Diastole:** The process of *chamber filling*.

   • *Atrial diastole* occurs as the right and left atria relax and blood flows into the atrial chambers from the vena cava and the pulmonary veins.

   • As pressure in the atria increases (secondary to increased volume) the atrioventricular (AV) valves (mitral and tricuspid) open, allowing blood to flow into the ventricles.

   • This process is known as *ventricular diastole,* but is usually not a distinctly recognizable component of the cardiac cycle.

◆ **Systole:** the process of *chamber emptying*.
  • *Ventricular systole:* When the ventricles fill, the AV valves close and the ventricular muscle contracts, resulting in the opening of the 2 semilunar valves (pulmonic and aortic valves).
  • *Atrial kick* or *atrial systole* is the assistance in ventricular filling, augmented by contraction of the atrial muscle.

Cellular Respiration

■ Gas exchange at the cell level is a result of diffusion due to differences in concentration gradients.

■ O_2 diffuses from the blood into the tissues and carbon dioxide (CO_2) moves from the tissue into the blood.

■ The blood is then re-oxygenated through the cardiopulmonary system and the CO_2 is removed through the pulmonary and renal systems.

Factors Affecting Oxygenation

Age

■ Older Adults
  ◆ Loss of alveolar gas exchange and a decrease in the partial pressure of O_2.
  ◆ More susceptible to respiratory infections because of decreased cilia activity.

■ Infants
  ◆ Increased O_2 needs due to higher basal metabolic rate.
  ◆ More susceptible to respiratory infection because of short, small respiratory tract.

Environment & Lifestyle

■ Exposure to dust, animal dander, asbestos or toxic chemicals increases the risk for alterations in oxygenation.

■ Obesity can inhibit thorax cavity expansion.

■ Smoking and exposure to secondhand smoke can alter respiratory function and oxygenation status.

Diseases

■ **Obstructive Pulmonary Disease:** Alterations in ventilation related to obstruction or restriction.

◆ The end result is impaired exhalation, air trapping and difficulty bringing fresh air into the alveoli.

◆ Airways become partially or completely blocked, resulting in diminished airflow.

◆ Lungs lose their elastic recoil, trapping stale air (normally that air would be exhaled).

◆ Most common obstructive pulmonary diseases, collectively know as **COPD** (chronic obstructive pulmonary disease) are:
   • Asthma
   • Emphysema
   • Chronic bronchitis

■ **Restrictive Pulmonary Disease:** Impaired ability of the chest wall and/or lungs to expand during the inspiratory phase of ventilation, resulting in increased work of breathing and reduced airflow into the alveoli.

◆ Common causes of restrictive pulmonary disease are:
   • Pneumonia
   • Pulmonary fibrosis (scarring)
   • Traumatic injury to the thorax such as multiple rib fractures resulting in "flail chest" or paradoxical chest wall movement.
   • Pleural defects: Collection of fluid or air between the components of the respiratory anatomy.
   • Atelectasis: Alveolar collapse.

Diffusion Defects
■ A decrease in the efficiency of gas diffusion from the alveolar space into the pulmonary capillary blood.
■ Diffusion defects usually coexist with obstructive or restrictive pulmonary diseases.

Ventilation/Perfusion (V/P) Mismatching
■ The balance between ventilation and perfusion.
■ The amount of air entering the alveoli (alveolar ventilation) and the amount of blood flow to various regions of the pulmonary capillary network (perfusion) are impacted by the effects of gravity, as well as by positions.
■ However, healthy lung tissue is able to compensate by producing vasoconstriction or bronchoconstriction, as needed to better match ventilation and perfusion.
■ When disease states make this compensatory mechanism ineffective, some alveolar regions will be well ventilated but poorly perfused (dead space), while other areas are well perfused but poorly ventilated (shunting).
■ Conditions that cause V/P mismatching include:
  ◆ Alterations in circulation
    • Right-sided heart failure
    • Pulmonary hypertension
    • Embolus (blockage of a pulmonary artery)

Heart Failure
■ The heart is unable to pump enough blood to meet the metabolic needs of the body.
■ When blood backs up in the venous circulation, the resulting condition is called **congestive heart failure.**

■ The increased pressure of the blood in the engorged veins causes fluid to leak out of the associated capillary beds, causing edema in the tissue **(pulmonary edema)**.

Anemia

■ A deficiency of hemoglobin decreases the O_2-carrying capacity of the blood.

■ The anemic patient may have a normal SaO_2 (oxygen saturation) level, but continue to experience inadequate tissue oxygenation at the cellular level because of a decrease in the quantity of hemoglobin.

Physiological Responses to Reduced Oxygenation

■ **Increased O_2 Extraction:** The cells extract more O_2 from the arterial blood.

■ **Anaerobic Metabolism:** The normal use of glucose for cellular energy occurs via metabolic pathway using O_2 (aerobic metabolism). In the absence of O_2, many cells can use an alternate metabolic process (anaerobic metabolism) for short periods.

◆ However anaerobic metabolism yields less energy and results in the accumulation of acid by-products such as lactate, which upsets the chemical environment of the cell and induces the release of cell-damaging enzymes (lysosomal).

■ **Tissue Ischemia & Cell Death:** Prolonged O_2 deprivation **(hypoxia)** leads to cellular death.

◆ The destruction of tissues or organs as a result of O_2 deprivation is known as an **infarction.**

■ **CO_2 Transport & Excretion:** CO_2 is a natural by-product of metabolism.

■ In the lungs, CO_2 is released into the alveoli by diffusion and exits into the atmosphere as the person exhales.

■ In the body, CO_2 functions as an acid as it combines with water to produce carbonic acid.

■ The hydrogen ions that are liberated in this process stimulate the respiratory control centers to increase the rate and depth of breathing.

■ Thus, the increased production of CO_2 as a result of fever or exercise may increase ventilatory rate **(tachypnea)** and depth.

■ An elevated blood level of CO_2 **(hypercapnea)** indicates inadequate alveolar ventilation.

Nursing Care Responsibilities

■ Nursing care for the patient with an oxygenation alteration/variation is prioritized on the basis of the A-B-C format used in basic life support and by using Maslow's Hierarchy of Needs, which identifies **oxygenation** as a basic survival need.

■ Primary nursing diagnoses related to oxygenation status include:

◆ **Ineffective Airway Clearance:** The patient has difficulty maintaining a patent/open airway.
  • Possible Causes
    > Obstruction by the tongue
    > Obstruction by secretions due to excessive production or ineffective cough
    > Upper airway obstruction due to edema/swelling of the larynx or glottis
    > Obstruction of the tracheo-bonchus by foreign body aspiration
    > Partial occlusion of the airways by infection, inflammation, smooth muscle spasm, or compression by a mass

> Occlusion of the distal airways due to chronic changes associated with emphysema
- Assessment Data
  > Complaints of feeling short of breath (SOB), also called air hunger
  > Difficulty speaking due to inability to "catch" breath
  > Weak, ineffective cough
  > Rales/crackles or rhonchi/snores upon auscultation
  > Diminished breath sounds (complete obstruction results in absence of breath sound in obstructed area)

◆ **Ineffective Breathing Patterns:** The breathing pattern does not deliver adequate fresh air to the alveoli, resulting in chronic air hunger and muscle fatigue.
- Possible Causes
  > Central nervous system (CNS) disorders
  > Effects of anesthetics and narcotics
  > Brain stem lesions
  > Major abdominal or thoracic surgical procedure
  > Mobility restrictions
  > Neuromuscular disease
  > Spinal curvatures
- Assessment Data
  > Pattern of rapid, shallow respirations

◆ **Impaired Gas Exchange:** Adequate air is delivered to the alveoli, but adequate O_2 does not enter the arterial blood and/or CO_2 is not removed from the venous blood.
- Possible Causes
  > V/P mismatch

> Decreased alveolar-capillary surface area available for exchange

> Atelectasis or pneumonia resulting in shunting

- Assessment Data

> Measurement of O_2 and CO_2 content in the arterial blood gas

◆ **Ineffective Tissue Perfusion:** Impaired O_2 delivery to the tissue and body cells.

- Possible Causes

> Atherosclerosis

- Assessment Data

> Depends on the tissue involved, but a common finding is **PAIN**.

NURSING NOTES

Because oxygen intake is essential to human survival, the professional nurse ensures the patient's **proper oxygenation** or implements therapy plan if needed.

6 **Nutrition**

Nutrition

- The consumption of nutrients is necessary to support physiological activities of **digestion, absorption** and **metabolism**, and to maintain **homeostasis**.
- Nutrition is the process by which the body metabolizes and uses nutrients.
- The metabolism of nutrients plays a critical role in supplying the body with the needed substances to maintain internal homeostasis.
- Nutrients are classified into 3 groups:
  - ◆ **Energy Nutrients:** Release energy for maintenance of homeostasis.
  - ◆ **Organic Nutrients:** Build and maintain body tissues and regulate body processes.
  - ◆ **Inorganic Nutrients:** Provide a medium for chemical reactions, transport materials, maintain body temperature, promote bone formation, and conduct nerve impulses.
- While nutrition is important for healthy living and health maintenance, it takes on *added significance during periods of illness.*

Physiology of Nutrition

The physiological process of nutrition includes **digestion, absorption, metabolism** and **excretion**.

Digestion

■ The mechanical and chemical process that converts nutrients into a physically absorbable state.

■ The anatomical structures and functions of the digestive process are:

◆ **Mouth:** Prepares foodstuff for digestion by mastication.

◆ **Salivary Glands:** Release lubricating secretions that bind with food particles to facilitate swallowing.

◆ **Deglutition:** Swallowing of food, which begins in the mouth and continues in the **pharynx** and **esophagus.**

◆ **Relaxation:** Cessation of the activity of the **gastroesophageal constrictor** muscle allows food to enter the stomach.

◆ **Stomach & Small Intestines:** Are the sites of digestive activities.

◆ **Peristalsis:** Coordinated rhythmic contraction of the smooth muscle lining the intestines.

• Moves **chyme** (partially digested foodstuff) through the small intestines to the large intestines.

Absorption

■ The process by which the end products of digestion—simple sugars (monosaccharides), amino acids, fatty acids chains, vitamins, minerals and water—pass through the epithelial membranes of the intestines into the blood or lymph systems.

■ Most of absorption occurs in the **small intestine** through the process of **osmosis, diffusion** and **active transport.**

■ The main function of the **large intestine** is to **absorb water** and **collect dietary fiber** or the parts of food that cannot be digested and absorbed.

■ Dietary fiber absorbs water in the large intestines, promoting the formation of a soft, bulky stool that moves quickly through the large intestine.

Metabolism

■ The aggregation of all chemical reactions and processes in every body cell as they relate to the **distribution of nutrients** in the blood *after digestion*.

■ **Metabolic rate** refers to the rate of heat liberation during chemical reactions, expressed in units called **calories**.

  ◆ A calorie is the amount of heat required to raise the temperature of 1 gram of water one degree Celsius (1° C).

  ◆ The **BMR** (basal metabolic rate) refers to the energy needed to maintain essential physiological functions, such as respiration, circulation and muscle tone, when a person is at complete rest both physically and mentally.

Excretion

■ The removal of **waste products** through the **intestines** and **rectum.**

■ This is the final digestive process prior to bowel system elimination.

Factors Affecting Nutrition

Age

■ **Infants:** Have a high risk of nutritional imbalances because of their physiological development.

  ◆ Factors such as the infant's total body surface area, immature physiological development, and rapid rate of growth and development result in a high BMR.

■ **Children (ages 1 to 6):** Nutritional intake varies with growth rate, making eating habits erratic.

◆ Adequate levels of protein, vitamin D, calcium and phosphate are important to complement teeth eruption and an increase in muscle mass and bone density.

■ **Adolescence:** Another period of rapid growth, as well as sexual maturation.

◆ The influence of peer pressure and other emotional stressors may impact eating habits and overall nutritional status.

■ **Adults:** Growth stops and metabolism declines, thereby decreasing the need for high caloric intake.

◆ Structural and functional changes may put older adults at risk. However, the aging population is not a homogeneous group because people do not age physically at the same rate as they do chronologically.

Lifestyle

■ Eating is a social activity in most cultures. Food preferences are usually developed in childhood and modified throughout the life span.

■ Lifestyle nutritional behaviors often come from family practices and affect not only food related behaviors but also the individual's beliefs regarding health and wellness.

Ethnicity, Culture & Religious Practices

■ Dietary customs reflect the socialization and cultural patterns of ethnic groups.

■ Religious beliefs may dictate what types of foods are eaten and how they are to be prepared.

■ While the nurse cannot learn the nutritional behaviors of every ethnic group (and/or variations within groups, as well as individual choices), recognizing the need to comply with the patient's routine patterns of dietary intake and preparation is important.

Other Factors

- **Economics:** Fresh fruits and vegetables and lean meats can be expensive and are often substituted with products that tend to be low in protein and high in starch, which are more economical.
- **Gender:** Primarily related to stereotyping—i.e., males eat meat and potatoes while females eat salads.
- **Peer Pressure:** Especially prevalent among the adolescent population.
- **Stress, Depression and/or Alcohol Abuse:** Can alter eating habits and patterns.
- **Medications:** Can alter absorption and excretion, as well as altering the taste of food.
- **GI Disorders:** Conditions such as anorexia, bulimia, nausea, vomiting, diarrhea, constipation, discomfort and/or pain all can impact food preferences and consumption.

Nursing Care Responsibilities

Assessment of Nutritional Status

- Nurses are in a unique position to recognize alterations related to inadequate intake, disorders of digestion or absorption, and overeating.
- **Nutritional History**
  - ◆ **24-Hour Recall:** Requires the patient to identify everything consumed during the previous 24 hours.
    - It is easy and quick to perform, but patients may have inaccurate recall—especially regarding the quantity of intake.
  - ◆ **Food Frequency Questionnaire:** Gathers data related to the number of times per day, week or month that the patient eats a particular food.

- The nurse can focus the questions in order to obtain desired information on intake of a particular nutrient such as cholesterol or fat.
- This method can also be used to validate the accuracy of the 24-hour recall and to provide a more complete picture of foods consumed.

◆ **Food Record/Diary:** The patient records all foods consumed—including portion size—for a period of *3 consecutive days*.

◆ **Diet History:** Elicits detailed information regarding the patient's nutritional status, general health patterns, socioeconomic status and cultural background.

◆ **Physical Examination:** Physical findings can suggest a nutrient imbalance.
- Rapidly proliferating tissues—hair, nails, skin, eyes, lips, tongue—usually show evidence of nutritional deficiencies sooner than other tissues.

◆ **Intake & Output (I & O):** 24-hour monitoring of fluid status, along with obtaining daily weight.

◆ **Anthropometric Measurements:** Body weight, size and proportions provide insight into the patient's calorie/energy expenditure, balance, muscle mass, body fat, and protein reserves.
- **BMI (body mass index):** Determines whether a person's weight is appropriate for his/her height.
  > A BMI of **27** or greater indicates **obesity**.
- **Skin fold measurements:** Indicate the amount of body fat. A special caliper is used to measure skin folds.

- **Mid-upper arm circumference:** An index for skeletal muscle mass and protein reserves.
- **Abdominal girth measurement:** An index of abdominal distension.

◆ **Diagnostic & Laboratory Data**
- **Serum albumin:** Plays a role in fluid and electrolyte balance, as well as in the transport of nutrients, hormones and medications.
- **Serum transferrin:** A blood protein, in combination with iron, that has a role in the transport of iron throughout the body and to the cells.

  > A sensitive indicator of protein deficiency.
- **Hemoglobin level:** Measures the oxygen- and iron-carrying capacity of the blood.
- **Total lymphocyte count:** An indirect measurement of protein depletion.
- **Nitrogen balance (BUN):** The degree to which protein is being depleted or replaced in the body.
- **Urine creatinine excretion:** Skeletal muscle metabolism leads to an increased release of creatinine. Measurement of the total amount of creatinine is an indicator of muscle metabolism. (NOTE: *Obtained by testing urine, not blood.*)

Nursing Diagnoses

■ **Imbalanced Nutrition:** *Less than* body requirements.
- ◆ A state when the patient is unable to ingest/digest food or absorb nutrients.

■ **Imbalanced Nutrition:** *More than* body requirements.

◆ A state when the patient's intake of nutrients exceeds his/her metabolic needs.

Diet Therapy

■ Therapeutic nutrition requires consideration of the patient's total needs:
  ◆ Cultural
  ◆ Socioeconomic
  ◆ Psychological
  ◆ Physiological

■ Nurses need a solid comprehension of diet therapy in order to assist the patient in making lifestyle adaptations and informed choices.

  ◆ **NPO (*Non per os* – nothing by mouth):** A type of diet modification, as well as a fluid restriction.
    • This intervention is ordered prior to surgery and/or certain diagnostic procedures in order to rest the GI tract.
    • And also when the source of the patient's nutritional problem is unidentified.

  ◆ **Clear Liquid Diet:** Consists of liquids that have NO residue, such as water, apple juice and gelatin. *Dairy products are not allowed.*

  ◆ **Liquid or Full-Liquid Diet:** Consists of substances that are liquid at room temperature (i.e., ice cream, pudding).

  ◆ **Soft Diet:** Promotes mechanical digestion of foods.
    • Used for patients experiencing difficulty in chewing or swallowing, or with impaired digestion and/or absorption.
    • Foods to be avoided include: nuts, seeds (including tomatoes or berries with seeds), raw fruits and vegetables, fried foods, and whole grains.

◆ **Low-Residue Diet:** Reduced fiber and cellulose, prescribed to decrease GI mucosal irritation.
  • Foods to be avoided are raw fruits (except bananas), vegetables, seeds, plant fiber, and whole grains.
  • Dairy products are limited to 2 servings per day.
◆ **High-Fiber Diet:** Food content that is high in fiber and cellulose in order to increase the forward motion of indigestible wastes through the colon.
◆ **Sodium-Restricted Diet:** Used with patients who have an excess fluid volume, hypertension, heart failure, myocardial infarction and/or renal failure.
  • Sodium intake may be restricted as follows:
    > mild: 2,000–3,000 mg
    > moderate: 1,000 mg
    > strict: 500 mg

NURSING NOTES
Nutrition is a vital process of the human body. The professional nurse strives to ensure the patient's adequate nutrition—**intake, digestion, absorption, metabolism, excretion**—including intervention therapy when diagnosis indicates that it is necessary.

7 Neuromuscular Needs & Care

NURSING NOTES

The nurse knows that the well-being of an individual is dependent on the functions of **sensation, perception** and **cognition,** because it is through these mechanisms that the person fully experiences and interacts with the environment.

Sensation

- The ability to receive and process stimuli through the sensory organs.
- There are 2 types of stimuli: external and internal.
  - ◆ External stimuli are received and processed through the 5 senses:
    - Sight (visual)
    - Sound (auditory)
    - Smell (olfactory)
    - Taste (gustatory)
    - Touch (tactile)
  - ◆ Internal stimuli are received and processed through kinesthetic and visceral modes.

Perception

- The ability to experience, recognize, organize and interpret sensory stimuli.

■ **Sensory Perception:** The ability to receive sensory impressions and, through cortical association, relate the stimuli to past experiences, thereby forming an impression of the nature of the stimuli.

Cognition

■ The intellectual ability to think is closely associated with perception.

■ Cognition includes the elements of memory, judgment and orientation.

Physiology of Sensation, Perception & Cognition

■ Sensation, perception and cognition are neurological functions.

■ The neurological (nervous) system is composed of 2 subsystems:

  ◆ **CNS** (central nervous system)

  ◆ **PNS** (peripheral nervous system)

■ The CNS and PNS act together to accomplish 3 purposes:

  ◆ Collection of stimuli from the receptors at the end of the peripheral nerves.

  ◆ Transport of stimuli to the brain for integration and cognition processing.

  ◆ Conduction of responses to the stimuli from the brain to responsive motor centers in the body.

■ The **CNS** consists of the **brain** and the **spinal cord**, which are protected by the bony structures of the skull and vertebral column.

  ◆ The brain is composed of 3 basic structures:

    • **Cerebrum**

    • **Cerebellum**

    • **Brain Stem**

- The spinal cord links the advanced neurosensory mechanisms that occur in the brain to the rest of the body via a coordinated pathway of neurons.
■ Sensory perception involves the functions of both the **cranial** and **peripheral nerves**.
■ The cranial nerves arise from the structures of the brain and govern the movement and function of various muscles and nerves throughout the body.
■ The peripheral nerves, which comprise the PNS, connect the CNS to other parts of the body.

Components of Cognition

■ **Consciousness:** A state of awareness of self, others and the surrounding environment.
 ◆ **Arousal:** State of being prepared to act.
 ◆ **Awareness:** The capacity to perceive sensory impressions and to react appropriately through thoughts and actions.
 ◆ **Orientation:** The ability to be cognitively aroused, to attend to the environment and to recognize patterns.
■ **Memory**
 ◆ **Immediate Memory:** The retention of information for a specified and usually short period of time.
 ◆ **Recent Memory:** Events that have occurred in the past 24 hours.
 ◆ **Remote Memory:** The retention of experiences that occurred during an earlier period of life.
■ **Affect:** Mood or feeling that can impact thinking ability.
■ **Judgment:** The ability to compare or evaluate alternatives to life situations, ultimately arriving at an appropriate course of action.

Mobility

■ The ability to move and engage in activity promotes health and well-being, whereas immobility presents a threat to physical, mental and social well-being.

■ Mobility is the ability to engage in free movements, such as walking, sitting, standing, pushing, pulling, and performing activities of daily living (ADLs).

■ Mobility influences the functions of many body systems, such as the respiratory, GI and urinary systems, and enhances muscle tone and energy level.

■ **Body Alignment:** The position of body parts in relation to each other.

■ **Muscle Tone & Bone Strength:** Allow a person to maintain an erect posture.

■ Proper body alignment is characterized by:
   ◆ Head upright
   ◆ Face forward
   ◆ Shoulders square
   ◆ Back straight
   ◆ Abdominal muscles tucked in
   ◆ Arms straight at side
   ◆ Hands with palms forward
   ◆ Legs straight
   ◆ Feet forward

■ Muscle tone in a normal state of balanced tension allows a muscle to respond quickly to stimuli.
   ◆ Alterations in muscle tone include:
      • **Hypotonicity** (flaccidity): a decrease in muscle tone.
      • **Hypertonicity** (spasticity): an increase in muscle tone.

■ **Body Mechanics:** The purposeful and coordinated use of body parts and positions during activity.

■ Use of proper body mechanics:
   ◆ Maximizes the effectiveness of the efforts of musculoskeletal and neurological systems.
   ◆ Reduces the potential for harm and/or discomfort during movement.
   ◆ Prevents strain and injury to the muscles, joints, ligaments and tendons.

Physiology of Mobility

■ Mobility is controlled by the interaction of the **musculoskeletal** and **neurological** systems.

■ **Musculoskeletal System:** Function is to maintain body alignment and to facilitate mobility.

Component Anatomy of Musculoskeletal System

Bones	• Facilitate mobility. • Protect body structures. • Produce blood cells.
Joints	• Facilitate motion. • Allow flexibility.
Tendons	• Cause movement of muscles.
Ligaments	• Support and strengthen joints. • Facilitate mobility. • Protect structures.
Bursae	• Prevent friction between bones and cartilage. • Facilitate gliding of muscles/tendons over bony surfaces.
Cartilage	• Facilitates mobility.

■ **Neurological (Nervous) System:** Muscle contraction is regulated by the central nervous system (CNS).

◆ Nerve impulses stimulate the muscle to contract.

◆ The afferent pathways convey information from sensory receptors to the CNS.

◆ The efferent pathways transmit the desired response to skeletal muscles via the somatic nervous system.

◆ **Proprioception:** The awareness of posture, movement and changes in equilibrium, as well as the knowledge of position, weight and resistance of objects in relation to the body.

  • Nerve endings in muscles, tendons and joints (proprioceptors) continuously provide input to the brain, which in turn regulates smooth, coordinated involuntary movement.

◆ **Postural Reflexes:** Postural tonus is maintained by righting reflexes.

REFLEX	DESCRIPTION
Labyrinthine Sense	Sensory organs in the inner ear (labyrinth) activate impulses when the head is turned.
Tonic Neck Righting Reflexes	Affected by movement of head from side to side. Neck muscle tonus is affected most when neck is hyperextended.
Optic Reflex	Visual sensations affect posture by helping the person establish spatial relationships to surrounding objects.

REFLEX	DESCRIPTION
Kinesthetic Sense	Activated when nerve endings in muscles and tendons are stimulated by movement of the joints. Informs the brain of the location of a body part.
Extensor Reflex	When the extensor muscles are stretched beyond a certain point, their stimulation causes a reflex contraction that counteracts the gravitational pull.
Plantar Reflexes	Reflexive contraction of the extensor muscles of the lower legs in response to pressure against the sole of the foot by the floor or ground.

Factors Affecting Mobility

■ **Health Status:** Influences desire for exercise and activity tolerance.
  ◆ Physical factors interfering with mobility and exercise include:
    • Fatigue
    • Muscle cramping
    • Dyspnea
    • Neuromuscular or perceptual deficits
    • Chest pain
■ **Developmental Stage:** Age and physical growth influence mobility and activity.
■ **Environment:** The home and/or workplace can be considered "safe and mobility friendly" if free of hazards that can disrupt or endanger mobility and activity.

◆ A sedentary lifestyle can lead to muscle atrophy, weakened bones, and a lack of motivation and energy to engage in physical activity.

■ **Attitudes & Beliefs:** Views on exercise and activity are affected by one's culture and family.

Physiological Effects of Mobility & Immobility

Immobility affects a variety of body systems and functions:

Neurological	**Gastrointestinal (GI)**
• Sensory deprivation	• Decreased appetite
	• Stress ulcers
	• Constipation
	• Fecal impaction
Cardiovascular	**Urinary**
• Increased cardiac workload	• Urinary stasis
• Orthostatic hypotension	• Urinary tract infection (UTI)
• Formation of thrombus	• Calculi
Respiratory	**Integumentary**
• Increased respiratory effort	• Pressure ulcers
• Hypostatic pneumonic	• Skin shearing
• Altered gas exchange	
Musculoskeletal	**Psychological**
• Decreased bone density	• Anxiety
• Contractures	• Depression
• Muscle atrophy	• Helplessness, hopelessness
• Increased pain	• Increased dependency

Nursing Care Responsibilities

■ **Bed Rest:** A therapeutic intervention that provides rest for patients who are exhausted, decreases the body's oxygen consumption, and reduces pain and discomfort.

◆ However, bed rest can also be counterproductive—inactivity caused by bed rest causes structural changes in joints and shortens muscles.

◆ Changes such as decreased range of motion (ROM) and contractures can occur within 48 hours.

◆ Therefore, an important nursing responsibility is to *prevent immobility.*

◆ *Approximately 7 days are needed for the patient to regain the function lost during 1 day of bed rest.*

■ **Body Alignment:** When patients are unable to move independently, nurses are entrusted to use proper turning and positioning techniques in order to:

◆ Increase comfort.

◆ Prevent contractures.

◆ Prevent decubi (pressure or bed sores).

◆ Make portions of the body accessible for procedures.

◆ Help the patient to access his/her environment.

• If the patient is unable to move independently, he/she MUST be repositioned every 2 hours.

• When positioning a patient in bed, the hips should be even with the middle of the bed (between the knee elevation and the head elevation portions).

• 3 essential principles must be considered when positioning patients:

> **Pressure:** Compromises circulation and leads to skin breakdown and ulceration.
> **Friction:** Caused when the skin is dragged across a rough surface, such as bedsheets, stretchers or other surfaces.
> **Skin shear:** Tearing of the deep layers of skin as a result of being dragged across a hard surface.

■ **Range of Motion (ROM) Exercises:** During ROM exercises, each joint is taken through its full functional motion in order to help the patient:
◆ Maintain full flexibility.
◆ Maintain muscle tone and strength.
◆ Prevent contractures.
◆ Improve circulation.

NURSING NOTES

Mobility provides enormous physiological and psychological benefits to the patient. Even when bed rest is prescribed, the professional nurse is responsible for ensuring that the serious side effects of immobility do not set in. **Resumed mobility is always the primary goal.**

8 Skin Integrity & Healing

■ The skin is the body's largest organ.
  ◆ **Epidermis:** outer layer
  ◆ **Dermis:** inner layer

Wounds

A wound is any disruption of body tissue integrity.

Types of Wounds

■ **Acute:** An injury, such as a stab, gunshot or burn; or a surgical incision.
■ **Chronic:** A wound that fails to heal or recurs without a new injury to the area.
■ **Open:** A break in the skin tissue.
■ **Closed:** No break in the skin, but soft-tissue damage is evident.

Classification of Surgical Wounds

■ **Clean:** Closed surgical wound that did not enter the gastrointestinal (GI), respiratory or genitourinary system. *Risk of infection is low.*
■ **Clean/Contaminated:** Wound entering the GI, respiratory or genitourinary system. *Risk of infection is moderate.*
■ **Contaminated:** Open, traumatic wound or a surgical wound with a break in asepsis. *Risk of infection is high.*
■ **Infected:** Wound site with pathogens present. *Infection is present.*

Factors Affecting Skin Integrity

■ **Circulation:** Poor circulation leads to changes in skin color, texture, thickness, moisture and/or temperature, which can result in ulceration.

■ **Nutrition:** A deficiency in protein or calories leads to dry, flaky skin.

■ **Condition of Epidermis:** Abnormally dry or excessively moist skin can predispose to altered integrity.

■ **Infection:** Localized and/or systemic infections can affect skin integrity.

■ **Systemic Disease:** Many systemic diseases impact skin health.

■ **Trauma:** Wounds can damage the skin with both short- and long-term effects.

Causes of Skin Damage

■ **Friction:** Any instance of the skin rubbing against another surface, usually resulting in irritation.

■ **Shear:** Tissue layers moving on each other, causing the blood vessels in the cutaneous tissue to stretch.

■ **Pressure**: Intensity and duration of pressure in conjunction with tissue tolerance.

■ **Pressure Ulcer:** A localized area of tissue destruction caused by compression of the soft tissue.

■ **Compression** → decreased blood flow → impaired supply of oxygen and nutrients → cell death and decomposition → ulcer formation

Pressure Ulcer Staging

Stage I
- Non-blanching erythema with intact epidermis.
- Defines area of persistent redness or red/blue/purple color change.

Stage II
- Epidermis is broken.
- Lesion is superficial with partial-thickness skin loss.
- Begins as an abrasion, blister or shallow crater, which progresses to a painful ulcer.

Stage III
- Full-thickness skin loss through the dermis into subcutaneous tissue.
- Appearance is a deep crater.
- May require months to heal.

Stage IV
- Full-thickness skin loss extending into the supportive tissues, such as muscle, tendons and bone.
- Sinus tracts may develop.

Wound Dressings
- **Gauze Dressing:** Fills wound and absorbs drainage.
- **Transparent Dressing**: Occlusive to liquid and bacteria.
- **Composite Dressing:** Absorbs drainage and only needs to be changed 3 times a week.
- **Hydrocolloids:** Occlusive to microorganisms and liquids. Also promotes absorption of wound exudates and enhances autolysis of necrotic tissue within the wound bed.

- **Hydrogel:** Maintains an appropriately moist wound surface. Permeable to oxygen and can fill dead space in the wound.
- **Calcium Alginate:** Absorbs large quantities of drainage.

NURSING NOTES

Because the skin provides multiple **protective, sensory** and **regulatory** functions, the nurse ensures the patient's skin integrity. Particularly critical is the nurse's responsibility for *preventing infection in wounds*.

Blood Analysis

Blood Basics
- Blood work provides the nurse with key information about the state of a patient's health.
- Blood carries out many vital functions as it circulates through the body:
  - Transporting oxygen (O_2) from the lungs to other body tissues.
  - Carrying carbon dioxide (CO_2) away from body tissues.
  - Distributing nutrients from the digestive system to the cells of the body.
  - Carrying away wastes for excretion by the kidneys.
  - Helping the body fight off infectious agents.
  - Inactivating toxins.
  - Using its ability to clot to stop bleeding.
  - Regulating body temperature.

Hematology
- Hematology is the study of the blood, its composition and functions.
- Plasma is part of the body's extracellular fluids.
  - The average adult has approximately 3 liters of plasma.

Complete Blood Count (CBC)
- Blood test ordered to determine general health status and to screen for a variety of disorders, such as anemia and infection.

◆ **Red Blood Cells (RBCs):** Also called **erythro-cytes**, the RBCs carry O_2 from the lungs to the tissues and take CO_2 away.

　• **Hemoglobin**, found in RBCs, is a protein that binds oxygen. It is tested to measure the amount of oxygen-carrying protein in the blood.

　• **Hematocrit** measures the amount of space the RBCs take up in the blood. It is reported as a percentage.

◆ **White Blood Cells (WBCs):** Also called **leukocytes**, the WBCs help fight infection.

　• The WBC count is the actual number of white blood cells per volume of blood.

　• The **WBC differential** looks at the types of white blood cells present. There are 5 different types of white blood cells, each with its own function in protecting us from infection.

　　> **Neutrophils:** (also known as segs, PMNs, grans): Phagocytes that engulf bacteria and cellular debris. An increase in the number of neutrophils occurs in acute infections, certain malignant neoplastic diseases, and some other disorders.

　　> **Lymphocytes:** A granulocytic leukocyte (WBC) that normally makes up about 25% of the total WBC count but increases in the presence of infection. Lymphocytes occur in 2 forms:

　　　- **B cells:** The chief agents of the humoral immune system, B cells recognize specific antigens and produce antibodies against them.

　　　- **T cells:** The agents of the cell-mediated immune system, T cells secrete immuno-logically active compounds and assist B cells in their function.

> **Monocytes:** Type of granular leukocyte (WBC) that functions in the ingestion of bacteria and other foreign particles.

> **Eosinophils:** Leukocyte (WBC) readily stained with eosin. Eosinophils, normally about 1–3% of the total WBCs, are believed to function in allergic responses and in resisting some infections.

> **Basophils:** Type of leukocyte (WBC), with coarse granules that stain blue when exposed to a basic dye. Basophils normally constitute 1% or less of the total WBC count but may increase or decrease in certain diseases.

◆ **Platelets:** Help stop bleeding by forming a clot.
  • The platelet count is the number of platelets in a given volume of blood.

Blood Typing

■ A **blood type** (or **blood group**) arises owing to the presence of antigens of a particular molecular structure on the surface membrane of RBCs, which exist in different variants among members of the same species.

■ Classification of an individual's blood is given in terms of specific, distinctive antigenic characteristics that are inherited and are associated with the RBCs.

ABO Blood Type, Antigen & Antibodies

■ **Blood Type A:**
  ◆ **A antigens** on the **RBC** surface.
  ◆ *B antibodies* in the *plasma*.

■ **Blood Type B:**
  ◆ **B antigens** on the **RBC** surface.
  ◆ *A antibodies* in the *plasma*.

■ **Blood Type AB:**
  ◆ *Both* A *and* B **antigens** on the **RBC** surface.
  ◆ *No* antibodies in the *plasma.*
  ◆ **AB** is the **Universal Recipient.**
■ **Blood Type O:**
  ◆ *Neither* A *nor* B **antigens** on the **RBC** surface.
  ◆ *Both* A *and* B *antibodies* in the *plasma.*
  ◆ **O** is the **Universal Donor**.
■ **Rhesus System:** Blood transfusions between individuals of incompatible blood types can cause severe immunological reasons, including:
  ◆ Hemolysis
  ◆ Renal failure
  ◆ Shock

Blood Clotting

■ **Coagulation factors** are proteins that are essential for blood clot formation.
■ The **coagulation cascade** has 2 branches:
  ◆ If the damage is to **tissue**, the body responds by activating the *extrinsic* **pathway**.
  ◆ If the injury is to a **blood vessel wall**, the *intrinsic* **pathway** is activated.
■ Each of these pathways utilizes different coagulation factors, but both come together to *complete the clotting process* in the *common* **pathway**.
■ Normally, by the end of the common pathway, soluble fibrinogen (factor I) has been changed into insoluble fibrin threads, which have been cross linked to make a **fibrin net** and are stabilized at the injury site.
■ The threads adhere at this site, along with aggregated blood cell fragments called **platelets**, to form a **stable blood clot**.

◆ This barrier prevents additional blood loss and remains in place until the area has healed.

◆ When the clot is no longer needed, other factors are activated to dissolve and remove it.

■ The body's ability to stop bleeding may be determined by the bleeding time (in addition to a count of the number of platelets).

Blood Clotting Studies

■ Normal values may vary from lab to lab, so always check the values at your specific setting.

■ **Whole Blood Clotting Time:** 5ml of blood is placed in a glass container, kept at body temperature, and observed.

■ **Prothrombin Time (PT):** A blood test that measures how long it takes blood to clot.

■ **International Normalized Ratio (INR):** Many variables affect the prothrombin time, so all commercial **thromboplastins** are compared to an International Reference Preparation, which determines a **calibration value**, called an International Sensitivity Index, which in turn must be supplied with every batch of thromboplastin reagent.

■ **INR** = (patient's prothrombin time / laboratory's control prothrombin time)

■ **Partial Thromboplastin Time (PTT):** A blood test that measures the time it takes blood to clot.

■ **Fibrinogen Split Products (FSP):** A blood test that measures **fibrin degradation** products, which are caused by *clots dissolving in blood*.

■ **Thrombin Time (TT):** Thrombin is added to plasma, and the time taken to form a clot is recorded.

Blood Chemistry

■ Blood chemistry tests are performed on **serum plasma** (the portion of blood without cells).

Electrolytes

■ These ionized salts, found in blood or tissue fluids, are related to the fluid balance in cells.

■ When the element in an electrolyte is dissolved, it separates into ions (atoms or molecules that carry an electrical charge) and provides for a cellular reaction.

Electrolyte: Normal Value & Function	Increased Levels: Manifestations & Conditions	Decreased Levels: Manifestations & Conditions
Sodium (Na+) 135–145 mEq/L: Indicates the balance of salt and water, and the functioning of the kidneys and adrenal glands.	Increased pulse and BP, decreased cardiac contractility. Dry, sticky mucous membranes, flushed skin and thirst. Increased urine output, twitching, tremors, agitation and CNS irritability. **Medical Conditions:** Diarrhea, diabetes insipidus, primary aldosteronism, renal failure.	Bounding pulse, increased pulse. Pale, dry skin and mucous membranes, thirst, weakness, headache, confusion, seizures, abdominal cramps, anorexia, lethargy, dizziness. **Medical Conditions:** Heart failure, cirrhosis, nephrosis, massive diuretic therapy.
Potassium (K+) 3.5–5.3 mEq/L: Affects several major organs, including the heart. Potassium levels rise in kidney failure, and may be abnormal due to vomiting or diarrhea.	Irregular slow heart rate, decreased BP, ECG changes, possible cardiac arrest with extremely increased level. Increased bowel sounds, diarrhea, abdominal cramping and nausea.	Weak, thready pulse, shallow respirations, dyspnea, polyuria and nocturia. Decreased DTRs, muscle weakness, paresthesias, soft flabby muscles, fatigue, lethargy. **Medical Conditions:** Metabolic

Electrolyte: Normal Value & Function	Increased Levels: Manifestations & Conditions	Decreased Levels: Manifestations & Conditions
(Potassium [cont.])	**Medical Conditions:** Addison's disease, burns and massive trauma, metabolic and respiratory acidosis.	*(Medical Conditions [cont.])* alkalosis, primary aldosteronism, Cushing's disease, vomiting, gastric suctioning.
Chloride (Cl-) 95–105mEq/L: Levels often go up and down along with sodium levels. This is because sodium chloride, or common salt, is a major component of blood.	Deep rapid respirations, weakness, lethargy, respiratory depression. **Medical Conditions:** Metabolic and respiratory acidosis, dehydration.	Slow shallow respirations, muscle twitching and tremors. **Medical Conditions:** Prolonged vomiting and gastric suctioning, diarrhea, some diuretics.
Calcium (Ca++) 4.5-5.5 mEq/L or 9-11 mg/dl: Is essential to muscle contraction, oöcyte activation, building strong bones and teeth, blood clotting, nerve impulse transmission, regulating	Muscle weakness, increased fatigue, decreased DTRs. Hypoactive bowel sounds, N/V, constipation, anorexia. Personality changes, acute psychosis, bizarre behavior, lethargy, coma, cardiac arrest.	Tetany, (+) Chvostek's and Trousseau's sign, Increased DTR, largospasm, seizures, hyperactive bowel sounds, abdominal cramps and diarrhea. Depression, apprehension, confusion, delusions, hallucinations, memory impairment,

(Calcium [cont.]) heartbeat, and fluid balance within cells. A deficit can affect bone and tooth formation, while overretention can cause kidney stones. Vitamin D is needed to absorb calcium.	**Medical Conditions:** Hyperparathyroidism, bone catabolism, immobility.	anxiety, hypotension, decreased myocardial contractility, ECG changes, cardiac/respiratory arrest. Increased bleeding and bruising, dry brittle nails and hair. **Medical Conditions:** Crohn's disease, hyperphosphatemia, drugs (aminoglycosides, antiacids with aluminum, caffeine, cisplatin, corticosteroids, loop diuretics).
Magnesium (Mg++) 1.3–2.0 mEq/L: Is used in building bones, manufacturing proteins, releasing energy from muscle storage, and regulating body temperature.	Decreased DTRs, decreased neuromuscular activity, decreased BP, HR. Possible cardiac arrest, somnolence, weakness and lethargy, respiratory depression. Flushing and sensation of warmth. **Medical Conditions:** Chronic renal failure, acute adrenocortical insufficiency.	Muscle twitching and tremors, increased DTRs, convulsions and hallucinations. Supraventricular tachycardia, PVCs and V-Fib. **Medical Conditions:** Chronic diarrhea and alcoholism, steatorrhea, starvation, bowel resection, diuretics, hypoparathyroidism.

Electrolyte: Normal Value & Function	Increased Levels: Manifestations & Conditions	Decreased Levels: Manifestations & Conditions
Phosphate: (HPO⁻) 2.7–4.5 mg/dl: Is needed to build and repair bones and teeth, help nerves function, and make muscles contract.	Hypocalcemia, soft tissue calcification, ECG changes, increased pulse, muscle spasm and weakness. **Medical Conditions:** Renal insufficiency, blood transfusions, muscle necrosis, hypoparathyroidism.	Anemia, bleeding, bruising, slurred speech, confusion, muscle weakness, paresthesias, chest pain, dysrhythmias, heart failure and shock, alkalosis, hypoactive bowel sounds, anorexia, vomiting, gastric atony, ileus. **Medical Conditions:** Alcohol withdrawal, hyperventilation, diabetic ketoacidosis, phosphate-binding antiacids.

Blood Glucose

■ Measures the amount of glucose in the blood at the time of sample collection.

■ Blood glucose may be measured on the following bases:
  ◆ Fasting (collected after an 8- to 10-hour fast)
  ◆ Random (at any time)
  ◆ Postprandial (after a meal)

■ It can also be measured as part of an oral glucose tolerance test (OGTT/GTT).

Blood Enzymes

■ Enzymes are **proteins** that *catalyze* a chemical reaction within the cells.

■ Enzyme tests play a role in diagnosing the degree of tissue damage, because enzymes are released into the bloodstream in proportion to the degree of cellular damage.

■ **Troponin T & I:** Current guidelines from the American College of Cardiology Committee state that cardiac troponins are the preferred markers for detecting myocardial cell injury.

Enzyme	Normal	Onset	Peaks	Duration
Troponin T & I (TnT & TnI)	Not present in healthy persons: **TnT:** Less than 0.1 µg/L **TnI:** Less than 0.3 µg/L	Rises 2 to 6 hours after injury.	Peaks in 12 to 16 hours.	**TnT:** Stays elevated for 5 to 14 days. **TnI:** Stays elevated for 5 to 10 days.

■ **CPK-MB:** Found in large amounts in the heart muscle.

◆ A CPK-MB *greater than 3.0 ng/mL* may be present when there is muscle damage caused by a heart attack.

◆ An ongoing high level of CPK-MB levels after 3 days may mean that a heart attack is progressing and that more heart muscle is being damaged.

Enzyme	Normal	Onset	Peaks	Duration
CPK-MB	Less than 3.0 ng/mL (0% of total CPK)	4 to 6 hours	12 to 24 hours	Fall to normal levels within 3 days.

■ The enzymes **LDH** and **AST** are not specific to cardiac muscle injury and are no longer used in the diagnostic process for cardiac disease.

■ **Normal Results:** For adults, the normal range can be up to approximately 200 units per liter (U/L), but is usually found within 45–90 U/L. (NOTE: *Reference ranges for total LDH vary from laboratory to laboratory.*)

■ **AST (aspartate aminotransferase):** Enzyme released into the blood when certain organs or tissues (particularly the liver and heart) are injured.

■ The AST test measures these levels, aiding primarily in the diagnosis of liver disease.

■ Aspartate aminotransferase (AST) is also known as **serum glutamic oxaloacetic transaminase (SGOT).**

■ **Normal results:** For adults, normal ranges for the AST are laboratory-specific, but can range from 3–45 U/L.

Blood Lipids

■ This is the term for all the fatty substances in the blood, including: **HDL cholesterol, LDL cholesterol, triglycerides.**

■ **Cholesterol:** Essential to both the structure and function of the body's cells, cholesterol is an important component of cell membranes as well as a building block for certain types of hormones.

♦ **HDL:** High-density lipoprotein contains more protein than lipid.

♦ **LDL:** Low-density lipoprotein contains more lipid than protein.

♦ **Triglycerides:** Important to the transfer of the energy derived from food and into the body's cells.

Element	Optimal	Borderline	High Risk
Total Cholesterol	<200	200–239	>240
LDL Cholesterol	<100	130–159	160+
HDL Cholesterol	>60	35–45	<35
Triglycerides	<150	150–199	>200
Cholesterol to HDL Ratio	<4	5	>6

SOURCE: National Heart, Lung, and Blood Institute.

Arterial Blood Gas (ABG)

■ Measures the levels of oxygen (O_2) and carbon dioxide (CO_2) in the blood.

■ Evaluates the ability of the lungs to move O_2 into the blood and to remove CO_2 from the blood.

■ Specifically, ABG measures:

◆ **Partial pressure of oxygen (PaO$_2$):** The O$_2$ level indicates how well O$_2$ is able to move from the air space of the lungs into the blood.

◆ **Partial pressure of carbon dioxide (PaCO$_2$):** The CO$_2$ level indicates how well CO$_2$ is able to move out of the blood into the air space of the lungs and out of the body with exhaled air.

◆ **pH:** The pH is a measure of hydrogen ion (H$^+$) in blood, which indicates the acid or base (alkaline) nature of blood.

◆ A pH of less than 7 is acidic, and a pH greater than 7 is called basic (alkaline).

◆ The pH of blood is usually close to 7.4.

◆ **Bicarbonate (HCO$_3$):** Buffers are chemical substances that keep the pH of blood within a normal range. Bicarbonate is the most important buffer in the blood.

◆ **Oxygen content (O$_2$CT) & oxygen saturation (O$_2$Sat) values:** Like the PaO$_2$, these values provide information about the amount of O$_2$ in the blood.

◆ **Fraction of inhaled oxygen (FiO$_2$):** The concentration of O$_2$ being breathed.

◆ **A quick method of analysis:** Look at the pH first.
  • Draw an arrow if it is low or high.
  • An arrow indicating low (↓) means acidosis.
  • An arrow indicating high (↑) means alkalosis.
  • Next, look at the respiratory indicator (PaCO$_2$).
  • Draw an arrow if it is low or high.

◆ **Interpretation:** If the arrows are in the **opposite** direction, the problem is respiratory in nature—either respiratory acidosis or respiratory alkalosis.

- Next, look at the metabolic indicator (HCO_3). Draw an arrow if it is low or high.

◆ **Interpretation:** If the pH arrow and the metabolic arrow are in the **same** direction, the problem is metabolic in nature—either metabolic acidosis or metabolic alkalosis.

◆ **Additional analysis:** *Compensation* is present if the arrows of $PaCO_2$ and HCO_3 are opposite. *Partial compensation* is present if the arrows of $PaCO_2$ and HCO_3 point in the same direction.

ABGs—At Sea Level & Breathing Room Air

Partial pressure of oxygen **(PaO₂)**:	70–100 millimeters of mercury (mm Hg)
Partial pressure of carbon dioxide **(PaCO₂)**:	35–45 mm Hg
pH:	7.35–7.44
Bicarbonate **(HCO₃)**:	21–28 mEq/L
Oxygen content **(O₂CT)**:	15%–23% (15–23 mL per 100 mL of blood)
Oxygen saturation **(O₂Sat)**:	95%–100%
Fraction of inhaled oxygen **(FiO₂)**:	The concentration of O_2 being breathed is also reported—in fraction form.

NURSING NOTES

Much knowledge can be gained from clinical analyses of the blood, so it is essential for the nurse to ensure that the data from **blood tests** is accurately recorded and communicated to the health-care team, and that the patient is comfortable during the blood-testing procedures.

Also, it is frequently the nurse's responsibility to explain the blood work reports to the patient and to assist with any lifestyle changes that are required as a result.

10 Intravenous (IV) Therapy & Blood Transfusions

Intravenous (IV) Therapy

■ Supporting the patient's fluid and electrolyte needs is an integral aspect of nursing care.

■ The nurse has specific responsibilities related to IV therapy, including:
- ◆ Knowing why the therapy is prescribed.
- ◆ Documenting the patient's understanding.
- ◆ Assessing the patient for allergies to: tape, iodine, ointment or antibiotic preparations.
- ◆ Administering the fluid at the prescribed rate.
- ◆ Observing the patient.
- ◆ Documenting implementation of prescribed IV therapy in the patient's medical record.

Parenteral Fluids

■ IV solutions are sterile and packaged in plastic bags or glass containers. (Some solutions are incompatible with plastic or the molecules adhere to the plastic, necessitating the use of glass containers.)

■ **Crystalloids** are **electrolyte fluids** with the potential to form crystals and are used to replace concurrent losses of water, carbohydrates and electrolytes. [*See* chart on page 107.]

■ Parenteral fluids can also be **colloids** (nondiffusable substances) that function like plasma proteins in blood by exerting a colloidal pressure to replace intravascular volume only.

■ Examples of colloidal solutions are:

◆ **Albumin**
  • Increased albumin concentration results in fluid moving into the capillaries from the interstitial space.
  • Primary use is as a volume expander in the treatment of shock from surgery or trauma.

◆ **Dextran**
  • A glucose solution with colloidal activity that expands the plasma volume by pulling fluid from the interstitial to intravascular spaces.

◆ **Hetastrach (Hespan)**
  • A synthetic colloid that expands plasma and is used in treating shock caused by hemorrhage, burns and sepsis.

Managing IV Therapy

▧ General nursing care responsibilities for the patient with IV therapy include:
  ◆ Checking for correct solution.
  ◆ Monitoring amount and timing.
  ◆ Monitoring expiration dates of the IV system (tubing, solution, site and dressing).
  ◆ Being aware of safety factors.
  ◆ Ensuring patient comfort and correct positioning.

▧ Starting an IV line requires practice and focus, and should never be attempted without both.

▧ Discontinuation of IV therapy requires an equal degree of practice and focus.
  ◆ IV needles or catheters are removed smoothly (i.e., in alignment with the vascular structure).
  ◆ Pressure and a sterile dressing are applied to the site.

Tonicity	Example of Solution	Clinical Implications
Hypotonic	0.45% NS (Sodium Chloride)	Daily maintenance of body fluids and establishment of renal function.
	D5W (dextrose 5% in water)	Promotes rehydration of body fluids when less Na+ and Cl- are required.
Isotonic	Ringer's Lactate	Resembles the normal composition of blood serum and plasma. Potassium level is below the body's daily requirement.
	Normal Saline (0.9% NS)	Restores sodium chloride deficit and extracellular fluid volume.
Hypertonic	Dextrose 5% in 0.45% saline	Daily maintenance of body fluid and nutrition. Treatment for fluid volume deficit.
	D5 in Lactated Ringers	Resembles the normal composition of blood serum and plasma. Potassium level is below the body's daily requirement.

◆ The condition of the removed catheter and the site should be observed and documented in the patient's medical record.

▓ **Equipment:** IV equipment is sterile, disposable and pre-packaged.

◆ Visual inspection is done to evaluate the sterility of the equipment and to check the expiration date.

◆ Because IV therapy provides direct access to the intravascular system, the nurse uses aseptic technique and standard precautions when assembling and changing IV equipment.

◆ **Administration Set:** The plastic tubing that provides the infusion.

◆ There are several types of infusion sets:

• **Primary continuous infusion set:** Used to administer routine solutions that are ordered to infuse continuously over a 24-hour period.

• **Secondary infusion set:** Connected to the primary tubing at a connection site, this allows for the administration of a second solution, such as a medication. Also referred to as a **"piggyback."**

• **Primary intermittent infusion:** Delivers fluids/medications at prescribed intervals through an injection or access port.

• **Blood tubing administration set:** Specialized tubing with a filter used for the administration of blood.

◆ **Vascular Access:** Needles and short catheters provide access to the venous system.

• A variety of devices are available to complement the age and size of the patient and the type and duration of the therapy.

• As with any gauge needle: The larger the number, the smaller the lumen.

- **Butterfly** or **Wing-Tipped (Scalp) Needles**: Short beveled needles with plastic flaps.
  - > These needles are commonly used for short-term or intermittent therapy, for infants and children, and for adults with small veins or impeded blood flow.
- **Short Catheters:** Vary in length from 0.75 to 1.25 inches.
  - > **Intracath:** A plastic tube that is inserted into a vein.
  - > **Angiocatheter:** An intracath with a metal stylet to pierce the skin and vein.
- **Peripheral Intravenous or Saline Locks:** Devices used to establish a venous access route as a precautionary measure or for intermittent infusion therapy.
  - > A needle or intracath is inserted into the vein, and the hub is capped with a lock port (Luer Lock).

■ **Calculating IV Drip & Flow Rates**
  ◆ **Intravenous Flow Rate Calculation** (2 methods)
    - 2-Step Approach:
    - Step 1:   Amount of fluid divided by hours to administer = ml/hr
    - Step 2: $\dfrac{\text{ml/hr x gtts/ml (IV set)}}{60 \text{ min}} = \text{gtt/min}$
    - 1-Step Approach:
    - $\dfrac{\text{amount of fluid x drops/milliliter (IV set)}}{\text{hours to administer x minutes/hour (60)}}$
  ◆ There are also electronic infusion pumps to regulate IV flow rate.
  ◆ Conventional IV pumps can be set to deliver fluids or medications at any rate from 0.1 to 999 milliliters per hour.

■ **Common Problems Related to IV Therapy Administration**

◆ **Hypervolemia:** Increased circulating volume may occur from rapid IV fluid infusion.

  • This results in cardiac overload, pulmonary edema and cardiac failure.

  • The IV infusion rate should be monitored hourly as a preventive measure.

◆ **Infiltration:** The leaking of fluid or medication into the surrounding tissue.

  • The patient may complain of discomfort at the IV site (often the first sign). The nurse should inspect the site, palpate for swelling, and feel the temperature of the skin.

  • **Patients can be injured by IV infiltration.** Infiltration causes soft tissue edema, which can cause nerve compression injury with permanent loss of function.

  • If a **vesicant** (medication that causes blistering and tissue injury when it escapes into surrounding tissue) *infiltrates*, it may cause *significant tissue loss* with *permanent disfigurement and loss of function.*

◆ **Phlebitis:** Inflammation of the vascular structure.

◆ May result from either mechanical or chemical trauma.

  • **Mechanical trauma** is caused by inserting a device that is too large, using a vein that is too small or fragile, or leaving the device in place too long.

  • **Chemical trauma** may result from infusing solutions too rapidly, or from acidic solutions, hypertonic solutions and/or solutions containing electrolytes (especially potassium) or other medications.

◆ Listen to the patient's complaints of tenderness, which is the first sign of inflammation.

◆ Inspect the IV site for changes in skin color and temperature—warmth and swelling are indications of phlebitis. In many cases, a reddened or pink/red strip develops along the vein.

Blood Transfusions

The purpose of a blood transfusion is to replace blood loss with whole blood or blood components.

■ **Whole Blood:** Used to restore circulating blood volume in situations of severe hemorrhage.

■ Whole blood contains **red blood cells (RBCs), white blood cells (WBCs)** and **platelets** suspended in a fluid called **plasma**.

■ **Packed Red Blood Cells (PRBCs):** More commonly prescribed for transfusions than whole blood because they increase the oxygen-carrying capacity of the blood without the increase in volume (and therefore in cardiac workload).

■ RBCs contain **hemoglobin**, a complex iron-containing protein that carries oxygen throughout the body and gives blood its red color.

◆ The percentage of blood volume composed of RBCs is called the **hematocrit**.

■ There are about 1 billion RBCs in 2 to 3 drops of blood.

■ For every 600 RBCs, there are about 40 platelets and 1 WBC.

■ Manufactured in the bone marrow, RBCs are continuously being produced and broken down. They live for approximately 120 days in the circulatory system and are eventually removed by the spleen.

■ **Fresh or Frozen Plasma:** Plasma transfusions are ordered to replace deficient coagulation factors and/or to increase the intravascular components.

■ Plasma, which is 90% water, constitutes about 55% of blood volume.

■ Plasma contains **albumin** (the chief protein constituent), **fibrinogen** (responsible, in part, for the clotting of blood), **globulins** (including antibodies), and other clotting proteins.

■ **Platelets:** Transfusions of platelets are ordered to correct bleeding disorders (thrombocytopenia) by replacing platelets, which play a critical role in coagulation.

■ Platelets (or thrombocytes) are very small cellular components of blood that help the clotting process by sticking to the lining of blood vessels.

■ Platelets are made in the bone marrow and survive in the circulatory system for an average of 9 to 10 days before being removed from the body by the spleen.

■ The platelet is vital to life because it helps prevent massive blood loss resulting from trauma, as well as blood vessel leakage that would otherwise occur in the course of normal day-to-day activity.

■ **Cryoprecipitate:** Transfusion used to restore factor VIII and fibrinogen in the treatment of hemophilia A.

Nursing Care Responsibilities

■ Verify patient consent (some agencies have written consent forms).

■ Verify that the patient has an 18 or 19 gauge needle or catheter in the vein, and that it is patent.

■ Small gauge access devices will cause damage to the RBCs being infused.

■ Establish baseline vital signs (VS) and assessment data prior to initiating the blood transfusion.

◆ Temperature and presence of skin eruptions or rashes are of particular importance.

■ Check patient's blood type and identity against the label on the blood container and paperwork obtained from the blood bank.

◆ This procedure is complete by two RNs or an RN/MD as a double check of the correct patient and compatibility of the blood scheduled for infusion.

■ Use only normal saline (0.9% NS) with a blood product.

◆ Infusion with dextrose or lactated ringers can result in hemolysis and clumping of the RBCs during the infusion.

■ For the first 15 minutes after blood begins to enter the patient's system, closely observe the patient for a transfusion reaction. VS are usually taken at least every 15 minutes for the first hour, and then once every hour for the duration of the transfusion. (This entire step is repeated from start to finish every time a new bag of blood/blood product is hung.)

■ **At the first sign of a transfusion reaction: <u>Stop the blood infusion,</u> *but maintain the vascular access with the saline infusion.***

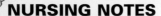

NURSING NOTES

IV therapy and **blood transfusions** are an integral aspect of nursing care, particularly in a hospital, hospice or nursing-home facility.

The nurse must display competence in the administration of these therapies, as well as in the monitoring of vital signs during such administrations.

Of course, the nurse is also responsible for the **patient's comfort** during therapy and for adding all documentation to the **patient's medical record.**

11 Medication Administration

Pharmacokinetics

Absorption

■ The rate and degree of passage of the drug from the site of administration into the bloodstream, **absorption** is dependent on several factors, including:
- ◆ The drug's physiochemical effects
- ◆ Its dosage form
- ◆ The route of administration
- ◆ Interaction with other substances
- ◆ Individual patient characteristics

Distribution

■ The movement of the drug from the blood to body fluids and tissues is called **distribution.**

■ The speed in which a drug reaches the tissue and organs depends on cardiac output (blood flow).

■ To reach the tissue, the drug must cross the cell membrane, but some membranes are barriers to medication distribution.
- ◆ For example, the **blood/brain barrier** allows only fat-soluble medications to pass through it and into the tissues.

Metabolism

■ The physical and chemical processing of the drug is a function of the **metabolism.**

■ In this process, the drug is inactivated and changed

into a water-soluble compound that can be excreted from the body.

■ The liver is a primary site of drug metabolism.

Excretion

■ The process by which drugs are eliminated from the body is known as **excretion.**

■ Excretion occurs primarily through the hepatic (liver) metabolism and renal (kidney) excretion.

Drug Action

Preparation & Route

■ Drugs are available in many forms and are prepared according to the form prescribed.

■ The route of administration refers to how the drug is absorbed.

■ Therefore, drugs prescribed for administration in one route should not be substituted with another drug form or route of administration without consultation with other members of the health-care team.

■ In addition, the nurse must be aware that certain forms of a drug require special administration techniques. For example:

◆ **Chewable tablets** are designed to be chewed before swallowing to aid in absorption.

◆ **Buccal** or **sublingual medication** must completely dissolve before the patient can drink or eat.

◆ **Suspensions** or **emulsions** should be administered immediately after shaking and pouring from the container.

■ **Oral/Gastric Route:** This route is the safest, most convenient and least expensive method. The disadvantage is that it is the slowest acting, as compared with other administration routes.

◆ The oral route is not used with patients who have GI intolerance (e.g., nausea and vomiting), are unconscious, or who have an order of NPO (nothing by mouth).

◆ Oral-route drugs are usually absorbed through the GI tract.

■ **Buccal** or **Sublingual Route**: The buccal (cheek) or sublingual (under the tongue) routes are used for rapid absorption of small amounts of a drug.

◆ Absorption is quicker because of the oral mucosal's thin epithelium and large vascular structures, which allow the drug to quickly be absorbed by the blood.

■ **Parenteral Route:** Injection of a medication into a body tissue. Sterile technique is always used for medication injections. The 4 routes that are commonly used for parenteral medications are:

◆ **Intradermal (ID):** Injection into the dermis.

◆ **Subcutaneous (SC or SQ):** Injection into the subcutaneous tissues.

◆ **Intramuscular (IM):** Injection into the muscle tissue.

  • **Intramuscular Injection Sites**
    > **Mid-Deltoid Area:** The recommended boundaries of the injection area form a rectangle bounded by the lower edge of the acromion process on the top to a point on the lateral side of the arm opposite the axilla (armpit) on the bottom. Avoid the acromion and humerus, as well as the brachial veins and arteries. Limit the number of injections here

as the area is small and cannot tolerate repeated injections or large quantities of medications >1 ml.

> **Ventrogluteal Area:** A good site as it is removed from major nerves and vascular structures. Palpate to find the greater trochanter, the anterior superior iliac spine and the iliac crest. When injecting into the left side of the patient, place the palm of the right hand on the greater trochanter and the index finger on the anterior superior iliac spine. Spread the middle finger posteriorly away from the index finger as far as possible along the iliac crest, as shown in the drawing. A "V" space or triangle between the index and middle finger is formed. The injection is made in the center of the triangle with the needle directed slightly upward toward the crest of the ilium. (When injecting into the right side of the patient, use your left hand for placement).

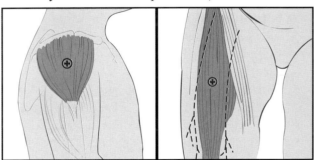

> **Vastus Lateralis Area:** A relatively safe injection site free from major nerves and blood vessels. This injection area is bounded by the mid-anterior thigh on the front of the leg, the mid-lateral thigh on the side, a hand's breadth

below the greater trochanter of the femur at the proximal end and another hand's breadth above the knee at the distal end.

> **Z-Track Technique:** A Z-track technique is used for administering any irritating fluid to "seal" medication in the muscle. Retract the tissue, insert the needle, administer medication, remove the needle, and release tissue. After injecting, note the tissue relationships resulting from the angled Z-tract left by the needle.

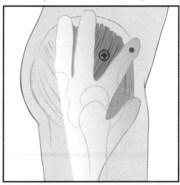

◆ **Intravenous (IV):** Injection into a vein.

■ The parenteral routes also include intrathecal or intraspinal, intracardiac, intrapleural, intra-arterial and intra-articular.

■ **Topical Route:** Given to deliver a drug at or immediately beneath the point of application. While most topical drugs are applied to the skin, other topical drug sites include the eye, ear, nose, throat, rectum and vagina.

◆ When applied to the skin, drugs are absorbed into the epidermal layer.

◆ Drug action varies with the vascularity of the skin, and most topical agents require several applications over a 24-hour period to cause the desired therapeutic effect.

◆ **Transdermal patches** are used to deliver medications for absorption into the bloodstream to produce systemic effects.

◆ **Eye, ear & nose drops** and **vaginal & rectal suppositories** are applied directly to the mucous membranes and absorbed into the bloodstream.

■ **Inhalants:** Are delivered into the alveoli of the lungs and absorbed immediately into the systemic circulation.

◆ Inhalants, including oxygen and most general anesthetic gases, are rapidly absorbed due to the permeability of the alveolar and vascular epithelia, abundant blood flow, and a large surface area for absorption.

Nursing Care Responsibilities

■ The process begins when a health-care provider writes a medication order.

■ The nurse is responsible for checking that the medication order is complete.

◆ A complete medical order includes 7 components:

• The name of the health-care provider who ordered the medication.
• The date and time of the order.
• The name of the medication.
• The dosage and frequency.
• The route of administration.
• The patient's name.
• The patient's identifying information.

■ Nurses have specific knowledge and skills that qualify them to administer medications and to evaluate a medication's effectiveness.

■ Nurses understand why particular medications are ordered for patients, as well as the physiological changes that are expected to result from intake of these medications, which in turn cause a therapeutic effect.

■ Because of their knowledge and skill, nurses can readily assess changes in the patient's condition, and, therefore, can determine whether it is appropriate to administer a medication based on the patient's current status.

Types of Medication Orders

STAT Orders	A single dose of a medication to be given immediately. The nurse needs to assess and document the patient's response to all STAT medications.
Single-Dose Orders	One-time medications. The nurse should administer these single-dose orders at the time specified. These drugs are often prescribed in preparation for a diagnostic procedure.
Standing Orders	Administered routinely as specified until the order is cancelled by another order or the prescribed number of days or doses has passed. The purpose of standing orders is to maintain the desired blood level of the medication.

Types of Medication Orders

PRN Orders	Administered on an "as needed" basis as circumstances indicate. Before administering a PRN medication, the nurse must completely assess the patient, using both objective and subjective data to determine the appropriateness of administering the medication. The assessment supporting administration of the PRN medication, as well as the patient's response, needs to be documented.

Safe Medication Administration

■ Nurses should administer medication in accordance with standards of safe nursing practice.

■ To protect patients from medications errors, nurses have traditionally used the "RIGHTS" of medication administration. (Traditionally, there were 5 RIGHTS; however, some newer sources are citing 7 RIGHTS, which are not listed here.)

The 5 Rights

RIGHT Drug

RIGHT Dose

RIGHT Patient

RIGHT Route

RIGHT Time

■ Routine medications are documented when they are prepared, whereas PRN medications are documented after they are administered.

■ If a patient refuses a medication, the nurse **MUST indicate** that the dose was missed, why it was missed, and that the nurse ensured follow-up with the prescribing health-care provider.

Dosage Calculations

■ There are 2 common methods that can be used to perform drug calculations:

Basic Formula: Frequently used to calculate drug dosages.

D/H x V = amount to give (x)

Fractional Equation

H/V = D/amount to give (x)

Cross multiply and solve for (x)

■ 3 elements are needed to use these formulas:
  ◆ **D** (**desired** dose)
  ◆ **H** (dose on **hand**)
  ◆ **V** (**vehicle**—form and amount in which drug is supplied; i.e., tablet or liquid)

■ *Remember: Before doing the calculation, convert units of measurement to 1 system.*

NURSING NOTES

The professional nurse employs a broad base of **knowledge**, along with critical **judgment** and an acquired **skill set**, in order to ensure that all medications are administered *accurately* and *safely*, so that the therapeutic effects are optimal.

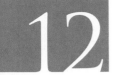

Caring in Nursing

- **The Focus of Nursing:** Nurturing people, caring, and growing by caring.
- **The Caring Moment:** Allows the nurse to truly experience nursing as caring, and to share that experience with the one nursed.
- **What Nurses Do:** Nurses enter into the world of the "other" (i.e., the one nursed) with the intention of knowing, affirming, supporting and celebrating others as both a caring person and a professional provider of care.

What Is Caring in Nursing?

- **Knowing the patient.**
  - ◆ Knowing and doing what the patient needs is fundamental to nursing.
  - ◆ The nurse engages with the patient in mutual problem solving in multiple areas of life—physical concerns, spiritual matters, relationships and family dynamics.
- **Having a presence with the patient.**
  - ◆ Letting each patient know that he/she matters is essential to nursing.
  - ◆ The nurse is present and available to the patient, and ensures the patient's awareness of and confidence in this presence and availability.
- **Doing for the patient.**
  - ◆ Responding to the patient's needs.

◆ Doing what the patient needs based on the nurse's knowledge and on the context of the individual nursing situation.

◆ It is important to note that doing for the patient sometimes involves unpleasant sensations (such as giving an injection, or getting a patient out of bed for the first time after surgery), but the doing is based on patterns of knowing and is in the best interest of the patient.

■ **Advocating for the patient.**

◆ Knowing when to stand up for the patient.

◆ First and foremost, the nurse protects the patient—protection is a cornerstone of providing care.

■ **Supporting the patient.**

◆ Providing a safe place for the patient and an environment in which the patient can get well and move to a higher level of well-being.

"Learning to nurse is essentially the process through which caring is affirmed, and professionalized through the acquisition of the cognitive, affective, technical and administrative skills specific to professional nursing practice." (Roach, M.S. *The Human Act of Caring.* Ottawa, Ontario: Canadian Hospital Association Press, 1984.)

NURSING NOTES

Technical knowledge
Level of skill
Caring
The professional nurse applies **"TLC"**—nursing style—with every patient, every time.